Caring for Depression

Caring for Depression

KENNETH B. WELLS
ROLAND STURM
CATHY D. SHERBOURNE
LISA S. MEREDITH

A RAND Study

HARVARD UNIVERSITY PRESS
Cambridge, Massachusetts
London, England

First Harvard University Press paperback edition, 1999

Library of Congress Cataloging-in-Publication Data

Caring for depression / Kenneth Wells . . . [et al.].
   p.   cm.
   "A RAND study."
   Includes bibliographical references and index.
   ISBN 0-674-09729-7 (cloth)
   ISBN 0-674-09730-0 (pbk.)
   1. Depression, Mental—Treatment—United States—Cost
effectiveness. 2. Depression, Mental—Patients—Medical care–
–United States—Cost effectiveness. I. Wells, Kenneth B., 1948–.
[DNLM: 1. National Study of Medical Care Outcomes (U.S.)
2. Depressive Disorder—therapy.   3. Depression—therapy.
4. Outcome Assessment (Health Care).   5. Quality Assurance, Health
Care. 6. Cost-Benefit Analysis. WM 171 C277 1996]
RC537.C274 1996
616.85'2706—dc20   96-4951

Contents

Preface

The private health care delivery system in the United States is rapidly changing, but little is known about the consequences for patients. This lack of data is particularly pronounced for patients with psychiatric disorders, and a cause of concern in a time when many insurers and employers limit mental health benefits and regulate the use of services.

As trends within the health care delivery system began to evolve, several private foundations and federal agencies funded the Medical Outcomes Study (MOS), a health care study involving more than twenty thousand patients and five hundred clinicians. Its purpose was to provide insight into differences in quality and outcomes of care in typical practices and to develop the tools to monitor outcomes. The Medical Outcomes Study was the first to include a psychiatric condition (depression) on equal footing with chronic medical conditions. No other study of depression thus far has been able to integrate clinical and health policies perspectives to a similar extent.

This book documents what we have learned about depression from the Medical Outcomes Study. Because it covers topics in epidemiology, clinical care, health services research, and cost-effectiveness analysis, we often refer the reader to journal articles for more details. Occasionally we expand on some methodological issues that we perceive to be particularly important or that are often misunderstood.

This book will be useful for a wide range of readers who may focus on selected chapters. Clinicians and educators will be interested in the information about the impact of depression on individuals and about key strengths and weaknesses of quality of care in the private sector, which may be helpful for clinician training, as well as to target quality improvement. These readers should focus on the introductory chapters (1–3) and the chapters providing clinical results (6–8). For health services researchers or managers in practices, insurance plans, or industry, our evaluation methods and measures of quality and outcomes should be of most interest. These readers should focus on Chapters 4 and 5 and the appendixes. Finally, readers interested in health care policy and policy research will find our cost-effectiveness work (Chapter 9) and discussion of policy implications (Chapter 10) to be most relevant, although this book is not a public policy book.

The Medical Outcomes Study and this book would not have been possible without support from the Robert Wood Johnson Foundation, the Henry J. Kaiser Family Foundation, the Pew Charitable Trusts, the Agency for Health Care Policy and Research, the National Institute of Mental Health, RAND, and the cooperation of participating health plans. The most important contributors, however, are the clinicians and patients who shared their experiences with us.

Caring for Depression

Chapter One

The Despair beyond Despair

Depression is more prevalent, causes more suffering, and has a more devastating impact on individual functioning and societal welfare than the public, policymakers, and even many health professionals realize. Patients with depression often withdraw socially, perform their usual tasks at work and home poorly—sometimes even stopping these activities completely and spending whole days in bed—and often think about suicide, the second most frequent cause of death among young adults.

The depth of suffering and the benefits of treatment have been powerfully described by the writer William Styron in *Darkness Visible:* "For those who have dwelt in depression's dark wood and known its inexplicable agony, their return from the abyss is not unlike the mythic ascent from Hell described by the poet Dante—a trudging upward and upward out of Hell's black depths and at last emerging into what he saw as 'the shining world.' There, whoever has been restored to health has almost always been restored to the capacity for serenity and joy, and this may be indemnity enough for having endured the despair beyond despair" (Styron, 1992). Yet many seriously depressed individuals receive no appropriate treatment for depression—even though depression can be treated successfully. Why is there such a discrepancy? Where does it occur and how can this situation be improved?

One reason for this discrepancy clearly is the continuing perception that depression is not a real illness. As a result, many people are hesitant to reveal their suffering to friends, family members, employers, and even their doctors, and are unlikely to receive appropriate care. There is little chance that this perception will change as long as there are no comparisons of depression with common medical conditions showing how serious depression really is. Such a comparison is one of the main goals of this book.

Because the quality of care for depression differs across delivery systems, we need to understand where problems are most likely to arise in order to remedy them. The quickly changing U.S. health care system offers a unique opportunity to make health care more efficient, but without information on health consequences, we will learn nothing about quality of care, and changes will be driven by cost-containment alone. An exclusive cost analysis misses half the picture—the half that patients care about the most. The integration of health outcomes and economic impacts in evaluating health care delivery is crucial to making policy decisions that benefit society.

The main changes in the delivery of health care in the United States are in financing strategies and managed care. Prepaid financing—which in the past meant health maintenance organizations (HMOs) but now includes many other organizational forms—alters patient and provider incentives to seek and deliver care. Managed-care strategies—such as gatekeeper policies—attempt to integrate management of a patient's overall health care, including mental health care. Although we do not know yet what these national trends mean for quality of care and health outcomes for all health conditions, this book provides a first detailed analysis for depression.

Such integrated health care evaluations will become more important in a competitive environment that requires information on costs and quality. Monitoring outcomes or quality of care for depression is not a trivial task, and using outcomes data to target quality improvement efforts or to anticipate the consequences of these efforts is even more difficult. We made much progress on these problems in our research over the past ten years. It is our hope that this book, by documenting our approach and measures of quality and outcomes of care for depression, will enable others to perform similar evaluations.

This book examines care for depression from a clinical view that depression is a major illness, in contrast with common usage, in which depression is an amorphous term loosely associated with "feeling blue" or being "down in the dumps." Clinical depression is a period of intense and often continuous feelings of sadness and hopelessness, accompanied by cognitive and somatic symptoms, that merits treatment. For those who have suffered from depression clinically defined, literature and medical experience testify that Styron's characterization of depression as "inexplicable agony" and "despair beyond despair" is not extreme.

Although there is disagreement among clinicians over what types of depression merit treatment, diagnostic systems distinguish several types. We focus on two: *major depressive disorder,* a severe episode of daily depressed mood accompanied by multiple symptoms such as suicidal thoughts or changes in weight and sleep patterns and lasting at least two weeks; and chronic depression, called *dysthymic disorder.* Dysthymic disorder has fewer symptoms but persists at least two years with only brief periods of respite. We also study patients with depressive symptoms that do not meet formal criteria for a depressive disorder because such *subthreshold depression* is very common in primary care settings. There are also bipolar mood disorders associated with periods of elation or excitement, called mania, but we do not study them here because they are rare and have different treatment implications than do depressive disorders without mania.

These different forms of depression raise different clinical treatment issues. Major depressive disorder is perhaps the best understood specific psychiatric condition, supported by many studies of treatment efficacy. Dysthymic disorder is a newer classification category and has fewer treatment efficacy studies. Subthreshold depression is little studied, and there is uncertainty about treatment.

Why Depression Is a Clinical Concern

Diagnosing depression is difficult because there is no obvious marker, like a spot on the skin or a blood pressure reading, and because depression can mimic symptoms of medical illnesses. Treatment for depression can be complicated in the presence of comorbid medical conditions, or if the patient already uses medications for other conditions. In general medicine, many clinicians cannot detect or treat depression in short visits of five to ten minutes that preclude attending to more than one or two of a patient's problems.

Patients who are otherwise similar often receive very different treatments depending on their type of provider. Clinical psychologists provide specialist assessment and psychotherapy, but they are not licensed to prescribe medications, whereas general medical clinicians rarely have the option to provide psychotherapy—even if they have the training and interest to provide it—owing to the constraints of scheduling practices in general medical settings. Only psychiatrists can easily provide both psychotropic medication and counseling, but this situation is changing under managed care, as the more expensive psychiatrists are reserved for medication management and consultation. These very different styles of care by specialty sector are likely to affect patient health outcomes and costs, which are central issues from both a patient and a health care policy perspective.

Why Depression Is a Policy Concern

Depression causes large economic losses because of increased mortality, morbidity, and treatment costs. In some ways, depression is worse than chronic medical conditions like arthritis and heart disease: those conditions usually strike later in life, but depression often begins in youth or middle age, when people are at their productive peak and thus are at risk of permanently damaging their careers. Depression also differs from many medical conditions because its indirect social costs (for example, losses from reduced productivity) are likely to be far higher than direct treatment costs. As a result, low rates of appropriate treatment for depression may be *socially* inefficient if increased treatment costs could be offset by reductions in indirect costs through better treatment.

Policy decisions about financing arrangements and the regulation of insurance systems can affect this tradeoff between direct treatment costs and indirect costs. Current debates often focus on the relative merits of different organizational and financial arrangements and how "generous" mental health care coverage should be. More generous mental health care coverage (low costs for patients, high reimbursement rates for providers) increases the probability that sick patients will receive appropriate services, but also the probability that other patients will receive services of little benefit. Because it is widely thought that the second type of error is more common for mental health than for physical problems, mental health coverage is typically lower than medical care coverage. Many employers offer special mental health and substance abuse plans that include intensive management and cost-control strategies. Mental health care has equal coverage with physical health conditions in some states with mandated mental health coverage, but then only for mental disorders that have a biological basis; this generally includes major depressive disorder, but not dysthymic disorder or subthreshold depression.

Most current trends in financing and organization of health care delivery result in reduced intensity of services. Many hope that this leads to more cost-effective treatment because the link between intensity and quality of care is weak. But these strategies could have stronger adverse effects on a condition like depression than on other medical conditions. Shifts toward primary care, for example, could result in fewer depressed patients being appropriately diagnosed and treated because primary care providers are less familiar with mental health conditions. Depressed patients could also be less capable of dealing with bureaucratic hurdles than other patients. Thus depression is an important test case for how general trends in health care delivery affect vulnerable patient populations.

How We Studied Care for Depression

Health care delivery systems are complex, and the multitudes of clinical conditions and treatments make it impossible to evaluate directly a health care system in its totality. One research and evaluation strategy to understand patient care is the tracer approach, which selects patients with specific health conditions. This approach allows us to go beyond typical policy in that we can study clinical details of quality of care.

Our empirical results are based on the Medical Outcomes Study (MOS), a four-year longitudinal study that involved more than twenty thousand patients with chronic conditions in different practice settings in Los Angeles, Boston, and Chicago. The MOS was one of the first large-scale studies to include a psychiatric tracer (depression) condition on equal footing with chronic medical tracer conditions (recent myocardial infarction, current congestive heart failure, hypertension, diabetes mellitus), and thus permitted a direct comparison of prevalence and societal impact across these conditions.

The Organization of This Book

This book is at the intersection of clinical, policy, health services, and economic research. We therefore first review the clinical aspects of depression and its impact on individuals (Chapter 2) and the policy context of studying care for depression (Chapter 3). We then discuss general design and analytic issues for evaluating health care systems (Chapter 4) and describe our measures of quality and outcomes of care for depression (Chapter 5).

The central findings of the MOS depression component are presented in Chapters 6–9. Chapter 6 documents the impact of depression on an individual's functioning and well-being; Chapter 7 discusses differences in quality of care and use of services by type of payment and provider specialty. Chapter 8 focuses on outcome differences, and Chapter 9 integrates these dimensions in a cost-effectiveness study of quality improvement and shifts to primary care. Chapter 10 concludes the main text of the book with a discussion of the implications of all our findings for clinical practice and health policy.

Because there has been much interest in measures of quality and outcomes of care for depression, and in the MOS measures in particular, we have included a technical appendix with key measures and scoring rules. Several tables with descriptive statistics provide a benchmark for other evaluations to compare their results with the MOS depressed patient sample.

Chapter Two

Depression and Its Treatment

Depression affects both individuals, by limiting their functioning, and society, by draining wealth from the economy. These are two complementary views of depression. The individual perspective is typical among clinicians and clinical research, whereas the societal is adopted in epidemiology and policy research. In this chapter we review the literature from the individual / clinical perspective: What is depression? How does it affect individuals? What causes depression and how can it be treated? How does this differ from actual treatment? In Chapter 3 we address the societal perspective: How common is depression? What are its social costs? How do policies on coverage, financing, and provider specialty affect treatment and social costs?

What Is Depression?

In the general and nontechnical sense of the word, depression consists of feelings of sadness or apathy accompanied by symptoms such as irritability, poor concentration, diminished or increased appetite, or loss of interest in activities usually enjoyed. Many people view depression and its symptoms as a continuum, from mild symptoms as part of normal daily life, for example, in response to an upsetting situation, to severe symptoms that can be persistent and disabling and require clinical intervention.

Prior to 1980, clinical formulations of depression distinguished between neurotic and psychotic and nonendogenous (response to an environmental stress) and endogenous (internally induced or biological) depression. These categories were not always defined operationally, and the validity of distinctions was not consistently supported empirically. In 1980, the American Psychiatric Association's Diagnostic and Statistical Manual, Third Edition (DSM-III), offered a new approach that represented a shift from classification based on etiology to a descriptive one based on identifying homogeneous conditions in terms of symptoms, course, and treatment response. Most subsequent disorder classification schemes followed this approach, which was based on empirical research and expert consensus. Such classification schemes are helpful for service delivery and research (Klerman, 1989b), but may best be viewed as a heuristic that identifies similar types of sickness. If the variation in terms of sickness and treatment response within a classification category is relatively large compared with the variation between categories, a classification scheme becomes less useful. Some argue that this has indeed happened, as psychological distress is a continuum and disorder schemes force arbitrary distinctions (Mirowsky and Ross, 1989).[1]

The two most commonly used psychiatric disorder classification schemes are the Diagnostic and Statistical Manual of Mental Disorders (DSM), now in its fourth edition (Task Force on DSM-IV, 1994), and the International Classification of Diseases, now in its tenth edition (ICD-10, World Health Organization, 1990). The ICD includes medical, surgical, and mental conditions and is used worldwide, including in the United States. Its codes and terms for psychiatric conditions are similar to those in DSM-IV.

Depression falls within the large category of mood disorders. We focus on the most common mood disorders, which in DSM-III (but not DSM-IV) were called unipolar affective disorders. Unipolar disorders involve periods of depression, but not mania. Mood disorders involving mania can be serious, but are much less common and are not discussed further in this book.

The most common mood disorder is major depressive disorder, which used to be called major depression. There is a small difference in the definition between DSM-III and DSM-IV, but seemingly minor differences in definitions can lead to different prevalence estimates (Philipp, Maier, and Delmo, 1991a, b). DSM-III, under which the MOS was designed, defines major depression as a period of at least two weeks during which an individual experiences daily disturbance in mood (intense feelings of sadness or loss of interest in activities that are usually pleasurable) and at least four out of eight symptoms: (1) too much or too little sleep; (2) appetite or weight disturbance; (3) psychomotor agitation or retardation; (4) loss of energy; (5) feelings of worthlessness or excessive guilt; (6) problems with concentration or indecisiveness; (7) loss of interest in sex; (8) recurrent suicidal thoughts or attempts. Major depressive disorder is not diagnosed if the syndrome is attributable to an acute grief reaction or a nonaffective psychotic condition such as schizophrenia. In DSM-IV these criteria were changed to the following: (1) symptoms must be present *most* of the day and nearly every day during the episode; (2) clinically significant distress or impairment in functioning must be present; (3) the syndrome must not be the result of the direct physiologic effects of a substance or a general medical condition; (4) major depressive disorder is still diagnosed after an acute grief reaction if the syndrome lasts for more than two months.

Major depressive episodes can also be associated with psychotic symptoms (delusions or hallucinations) and melancholia. Melancholia is characterized by loss of pleasure in usual activities plus at least three of the following symptoms: a depressed mood quality different from reaction to loss; depression worse in the morning; early morning awakening; marked psychomotor retardation or agitation; excessive guilt; and significant anorexia or weight loss.

About 50 percent of people suffering from major depressive disorder recover in a year, averaging across those receiving appropriate treatment and those not in treatment or receiving inappropriate treatment. The illness recurs in 50–70 percent of people who experience one episode, although many have one episode and never have a recurrence. Those with multiple prior episodes or chronic depression and those with comorbidities have worse clinical outcomes, which are typically described in terms of recurrence, time to relapse (exacerbation of symptoms before full recovery) or remission (recurrence of an episode after full recovery), and persistence of symptoms.[2]

The second common mood disorder is chronic depression, or dysthymic disorder.[3] Dysthymic disorder is a period of at least two years of depressed mood or loss of interest in pleasurable activities most days, although there may be spells of several days or weeks with few or even no depressive symptoms (Coryell, Endicott, and Keller, 1990). The DSM-III diagnosis also requires at least three out of thirteen symptoms, including symptoms of major depressive disorder (problems with sleep, energy, concentration, loss of interest, thoughts of death or suicide), plus other symptoms (problems with self-esteem, role and social functioning, irritability or anger, pessimism, and tearfulness or crying). DSM-IV criteria require mood disturbance as defined above, plus at least two of six symptoms (problems with appetite or weight, sleep, energy, self-esteem, concentration, and feelings of hopelessness) and evidence of clinically significant distress or functioning impairment.

Individuals can experience both major depressive and dysthymic disorders sequentially or simultaneously, which is referred to as *double depression* (Keller, Lavori, Endicott, Coryell, and Klerman, 1983; Keller, Lavori, Lewis, and Klerman, 1983). Double depression has a poorer prognosis than either condition alone, and recurrences of major depressive episodes are common. In this book, we refer to persons with major depressive, dysthymic disorder, or both as having "depressive disorder."

Historically, major depressive and dysthymic disorders were thought to account for most clinically significant depression. Recent studies, however, indicate a high prevalence of clinically significant depressive symptoms that do not meet major depressive or dysthymic disorder criteria. The terminology in the literature is inconsistent, referring to "minor depression," "subthreshold depression," or "brief depression." In DSM-III, these conditions could be classified as adjustment disorder with depressed mood, if they result from a specific stressful event, or atypical depression, but both categories are vaguely defined. DSM-IV added a category for "depressive disorders not otherwise specified" (depression NOS), defined broadly to include premenstrual mood disorders, minor depressive disorder (episodes of depression lasting two weeks or more but with fewer symptoms than major depressive disorder), recurrent brief depressive disorder (episodes lasting less than two weeks but occurring at least once a month for twelve months), and depressions related to psychotic disorders.

We will use the term "subthreshold depression" because the MOS used an empirically based (rather than clinical) definition. Patients were defined as having subthreshold depression if they exceeded a minimum score on the screener (see Appendix B) but did not have a current disorder. The minimum score was determined empirically to optimize the identification of patients with depressive disorders in the population, but it does not correspond exactly to a DSM category.

Practically, however, this definition of subthreshold depression is virtually identical to the mood disturbance criterion of major depressive or dysthymic disorder in the past year, plus recent symptoms. Among patients exceeding the screener, 50 percent of mental health specialty outpatients and 35 percent of general medical outpatients have a current depressive disorder.

Although these definition details may appear trivial, definitions can have surprising policy implications. In states such as California, Maine, and New Hampshire, for example, legislation identifies "biologically based" conditions that require parity with other medical and surgical conditions or must be included in health benefit packages. Included in such lists is major depressive disorder, but not other unipolar depressions. Similarly, an early version of Oregon's comprehensive state health plan that ordered conditions in their priority for reimbursement ranked major depression among the top one hundred disease conditions but ranked dysthymia much lower. Thus small differences in definitions can lead to dramatic changes in the incentives to seek and provide care.

Policies in turn are driven by the state of research. A disease condition is more likely to be considered for inclusion in a benefits package if its impact on individuals is clear and if there are proven treatments for it. In addition, policymakers tend to consider health problems with a biological basis to be more "real" than those without one. Research has provided strong evidence for a biological basis and for efficacious treatments for major depression, but there has been much less research on dysthymia or subthreshold depression, making the study of these conditions particularly important.

The Impact on Individuals: Mortality and Morbidity

Depression is the most common contributing factor to suicide, which can be especially tragic because serious depression is more common among young and middle-aged adults. Among patient samples with affective disorders, lifetime suicide rates are reported to be as high as 20–30 percent (Klerman, 1987). Thus management of suicidal ideation is a major focus in clinician training and treatment for depression. Depression may also be indirectly associated with mortality in that it contributes to the development of physical disorders such as cardiovascular disease (Rodin, Craven, and Littlefield, 1991). Overall, mortality among depressed persons is 1.5 times higher than in comparable demographic groups in the United States (Murphy et al., 1987).

Depression is also associated with morbidity, or limitations in daily functioning, including the ability to perform self-care tasks and household chores, and well-being, including emotional and social well-being. These impacts are especially important because depression affects young people with major role responsibilities (for example, childrearing, work). With the exception of social-role functioning, morbidity in depression has been a relatively unstudied area until recently (Broadhead et al., 1990; Johnson et al., 1992; Klerman, 1980; Ormel and Costa e Silva, 1995), yet physical functioning limitations could be as relevant for psychiatric conditions as for medical conditions: Wells, Golding, and Burnam (1988) found that a recent psychiatric disorder and a common chronic medical condition, such as arthritis, had similar correlations with bed days.

It is difficult to determine how much limitation in individual functioning or well-being is *caused* by a given disease condition, because many individuals have multiple health problems and because limitations in functioning can cause a secondary depression. This reverse causal direction, from limitations to developing a disease, is unlikely in medical conditions such as heart disease or diabetes, although there can be indirect effects if functioning limitations lead to behaviors that increase health risk, such as smoking, drinking, or overeating.

One way to determine causality is to compare whether or not treatment for depression improves functioning. Mintz et al. (1992) found that work functioning appears to improve with treatment of major depression, and Von Korff et al. (1992) and Ormel et al. (1993) reported reduced morbidity among psychologically distressed primary care patients as clinical status improved. Nevertheless, the causal effect of depression on morbidity is not yet understood. Although no one approach can unambiguously provide an answer (Von Korff and Simon, 1994), such information is important in calculating the social costs of depression compared with other medical conditions. The results presented in this book provide estimates of the association of various forms of depression with morbidity, while controlling for confounding effects of medical comorbidities, and compare these estimates with the effects of selected chronic medical conditions.

What Causes Depression?

Scientific theories fall into two broad groups: psychological theories, typically associated with advocates of psychotherapy, and biological theories, associated with advocates of somatic treatments. Neither type of theory explicitly addresses the other, but they are not mutually exclusive and actually complement each other. For example, genetic predispositions and life events can interact (Kendler et al., 1995), and biological characteristics can affect the response to psychotherapy (Simons et al., 1995).

At the moment, however, different clinical specialties remain associated with different theories, and professional organizations often use theoretical concerns to legitimize their opposition to policy changes affecting their economic position. With proposed legislation (strongly contested by physician groups) to provide psychologists with prescribing privileges and with changes in coverage favoring short-term over long-term psychotherapies regardless of specialty, the incentives for maintaining these different theoretical and treatment distinctions could change toward a more integrated biological and cognitive / behavioral orientation across specialties. In this respect, policy can change theoretical orientations and treatment preferences.

Psychological Theories

The most common alternative psychological theories of depression are directly associated with different schools of psychological treatment or psychotherapy.

Cognitive theories assume that cognitive activities, especially information-processing functions such as stimulus recognition and recall and problem solving, determine depressive symptoms. Aaron Beck (1967a, b) suggested that stressful events activate negative cognitive schemas, or long-standing perspectives that guide the interpretation of data. This results in information-processing errors, such as selective attention to unrepresentative data, drawing conclusions from inadequate data, and overgeneralization. When such errors become habitual, the resulting pattern of sustained negative affective and behavioral responses leads to depression. An alternative cognitive theory is "learned helplessness," derived from animal studies in which inescapable noxious stimuli lead to an automatic "helplessness" response, or no attempt to escape. Seligman (1975) suggested that depression in humans is caused by cognitive, motivational, and affective deficits that result from repeated exposure to uncontrollable outcomes.

These theories were the basis for cognitive treatments, such as Beck's cognitive therapy, which alter negative cognitions to eliminate affective and behavioral depressive symptoms. The effectiveness of cognitive therapy is indirect evidence for the underlying theory, but the scientific evidence for cognitive theories otherwise relies on the correlation between depression and negative cognition (Haas and Fitzgibbon, 1989).

Behavioral theories assume that depression is a learned response to the environment through reinforcement and conditioning. Poor social skills may lead to negative social interactions that reinforce low self-esteem. Behavioral therapies for depression are based on principles of operant and classical conditioning, that is, manipulating the environment to reinforce or extinguish behaviors. Manualized brief behavioral therapies have been developed using the techniques of activity scheduling, self-control therapy, social skills training, and problem solving (Depression Guidelines Panel, 1993b). As with cognitive theories, the efficacy of behavioral therapies provides indirect evidence for the theory.

The *interpersonal theory* of depression postulates that real or perceived losses activate depression in persons with undue interpersonal dependency, which may result from early childhood losses, disturbed intrafamilial relationships, or genetic or biological predisposing factors (Klerman, 1989a). Ongoing disturbances in interpersonal relationships maintain primary depressive symptoms. The interpersonal theory emerged from empirical research on hypotheses that stressful life circumstances precipitate depression and that social supports can reduce depression and buffer individuals against negative impacts. The evidence has primarily been from cross-sectional studies showing that depressed individuals report a high number of prior life stresses, but so do persons with many other psychiatric and chronic medical illnesses. There is also a significant relationship between poor social support and depression, even though the direction of causality is unclear. The relationship among stressful events, social support, and depression continues to be an active research area, but progress will require carefully designed longitudinal studies (Paykel and Cooper, 1992).

Interpersonal psychotherapy is aimed at mitigating the impact of current life circumstances and interpersonal relationships, not at underlying personality problems, and is efficacious for treating depression. The central goals are to resolve issues related to grief, role disputes, role transitions, and interpersonal deficits (for example, social isolation) (Klerman and Weissman, 1993).

Psychodynamic theories of depression emphasize the psychological meaning, consciously and unconsciously, of loss, whether of relationships, opportunities, or self-esteem, and the relationship of current loss to early childhood experience. Reviews of relevant theories can be found in Kelly and Cooper, 1989, and Mendelson, 1992. Different theorists emphasize different meanings or kinds of loss or have differing explanations for the sequence of intrapsychic events or conflicts that link loss to depressive symptoms. For example, Freud postulated that unconscious ambivalence toward a loved one resulted in hostility directed toward the self (Freud, 1917). Other theorists emphasized drives or instincts, for example, fixation of libido at the oral stage in response to frustration or disappointments in childhood (Abraham, 1948); narcissistic vulnerability to guilt and low self-esteem as a mechanism to restore love or acceptance (Rado, 1928); internalized "objects" or persons unconsciously identified as part of the self, such that rejection or loss is experienced as loss of part of the self, leading to depression (Fenichel, 1945); or regression to an infantile response to separation, owing to deficiencies in early bonding experiences (Klein, 1948). More recent psychoanalytic theorists emphasize the central role of self-esteem and internalized aggression in response to multiple environmental and internal factors (Jacobson, 1941).

Psychodynamic therapies are aimed at resolving unconscious conflicts through the therapeutic relationship, permitting new responses to emerge. Psychodynamic psychotherapies are typically long-term, but a manualized brief psychodynamic therapy has been developed. The efficacy of psychodynamic therapies has not been studied in controlled trials, however.

Biological Theories

Research has shown that depressive disorders are at least partly attributable to biological factors. Biological theories are based on research of different biological systems, but there is no integrated theory spanning different fields. Within each field, hypotheses often have inconsistent support across studies. In this respect, current biological theories have a more limited scope than psychological theories, but have been more directly empirically testable.

One prominent theory is the biogenic amine hypothesis, which claims that depression (and mania) can be attributed to abnormalities in neurotransmitter activity. Neurotransmitters are naturally produced peptides (biogenic amines) that relay impulses that activate or suppress a given neuronal pathway. Different pathways are associated with different specific neurotransmitters and brain functions. Abnormalities in transmission of two neurotransmitters, norepinephrine and serotonin, have been proposed as causes of depression (Caldecott-Hazard, Morgan, et al., 1991).[4] Reduced serotonergic activity is correlated with suicide attempts and other violent behaviors, but not exclusively among depressed patients (Caldecott-Hazard and Schneider, 1992). Transmission of other biogenic amines, particularly dopamine and gamma-aminobutyric acid (GABA), may be abnormal in major depression as well as mania (Willner, 1995). Evidence of the efficacy of tricyclic antidepressants, monoamine oxidase inhibitors (MAOIs), and selective serotonin reuptake inhibitors (SSRIs)—all of which affect neurotransmitter regulation—is consistent with the biogenic amine hypothesis.

Another biological function being investigated is secretion of neurohormones, a process regulated by the neurotransmitters hypothesized to be involved in depression. Diurnal variation in mood in some forms of depression, including melancholia, suggests disruptions in cortisol circadian secretion. This finding, together with hypersecretion of cortisol, is the most consistent result in neuroendocrine studies. Evidence of reduced pituitary secretion of adrenocorticotropic hormone (ACTH) in response to corticotropin-releasing hormone (CRH) in major depressives suggests that the abnormal cortisol secretion originates from the central nervous system—a finding that could potentially integrate neurotransmitter and endocrine abnormalities in depression. But these neuroendocrine abnormalities have been demonstrated mainly in depressed patients with melancholia, which has limited clinical applications of these findings.[5] Reduced secretion of thyroid-stimulating hormone (TSH) and growth hormone in response to various challenge agents has also been reported in smaller subgroups (about 20 percent) of severely depressed patients (Holsboer, 1995).

Sleep disorders are common in depression and may be another manifestation of abnormal biorhythm. Abnormalities of electrical activity in the brain during sleep, as measured through polysomnographic techniques, are among the most consistent biological markers of major depressive disorder. For example, about 60 percent of persons with major depressive disorder demonstrate a shortened latency period for onset of rapid-eye-movement (REM) sleep, which has also been observed in nondepressed first-degree relatives (Giles et al., 1989). Other abnormalities include heightened rates of REM activity and decreased sleep continuity (Kupfer and Reynolds, 1992). Sleep disturbances may be associated with supersensitivity of the cholinergic systems of the brain, but the precise relationship is unknown (Robbins et al., 1992).

Evidence of genetic risk for unipolar mood disorders further supports a biological view of depression. Family studies suggest that first-degree relatives of depressed persons are twice as likely to suffer from major depression as family members of nondepressed persons (Weissman and Klerman, 1992). The heterogeneity of depression limits the validity of genetic studies, and much of the literature only tries to identify homogeneous subtypes. There may be one family cluster for bipolar illness (bipolar depression and major depression in relatives) and one for major depression (major depression but not bipolar disorder among relatives), but even this pattern is debated (Gershon et al., 1989; Winokur et al., 1995).[6] Studies have been unsuccessful in identifying a specific gene map or linkage pattern for major depressive disorder, and there has been little research on dysthymia (Gershon et al., 1989; Weissman and Klerman, 1992).

Depressive symptoms or disorders can also be secondary to other psychiatric disorders, chronic medical illnesses, or a variety of medications such as antihypertensive medications. Hormonal disorders (hypo- or hyperthyroidism), infectious diseases (hepatitis, influenza), cancers, autoimmunue diseases, neurological disorders (Parkinson's disease, Alzheimer's disease), and other medical conditions can cause depressive symptoms. Some research groups have emphasized the importance of distinguishing depressions that are secondary to other illnesses from those that are "primary," because the course of illness and treatment implications differ (Grove and Andreasen, 1992). It is often difficult, however, to determine whether a comorbid medical or psychiatric illness is the underlying cause of depression or simply a concurrent illness.

Clinical Management and Treatment of Depression

Management Phases

Clinical management of major depressive disorder has four phases: (1) detection and assessment; (2) treatment of the acute phase; (3) continuation therapy for six months or more to prevent early relapse; and (4) ongoing maintenance therapy to prevent recurrence of an acute episode (Kupfer, 1991). The clinical practice guidelines for major depression in primary care include a whole volume on assessing depression type, severity, and presence of medical and psychiatric comorbidities (Depression Guidelines Panel, 1993a). Detection and assessment are a necessary step for treatment to be initiated, but detection alone does not have an independent effect on improving outcome (except for any effect that results from giving attention to patients).

For the other three treatment phases (acute care, continuation, and maintenance), clinical trials demonstrated the efficacy of various treatments. The efficacy literature is well developed for the acute care phase of major depression and for clinical symptoms, but short follow-up periods (six to eight weeks) in most acute care trials limit conclusions about long-term outcomes. Because treatment success in clinical trials is often defined as an improvement in clinical symptoms, not necessarily full recovery, there may be residual functioning limitations (such as an inability to work at a paying job) that, though they are rarely measured, would be very important from a policy perspective.

An important limitation in the efficacy literature is that depression types other than major depressive disorder have not yet been studied extensively. Many believe that treatments for major depression are efficacious for dysthymic disorder (Depression Guidelines Panel, 1993b), but establishing efficacy for dysthymic disorder requires long-term follow-up in treatment trials owing to the chronicity of symptoms. Trials of antidepressant medication and psychotherapy in subthreshold depression are currently under way, and one study suggests that cognitive therapy reduces subdiagnostic depressive symptoms (Miranda and Muñoz, 1994). Overall, the continuation and maintenance phases have not received the same attention as the acute care phase, especially for psychotherapy (American Psychiatric Association, 1993). Because there have been more successful clinical trials of somatic than of psychosocial treatments in all treatment phases, the AHCPR (Agency for Health Care Policy and Research) depression guidelines (based on prior research) have been perceived by some as medically biased and too unfavorable to psychotherapy (Muñoz et al., 1994), reflecting the ongoing schism between psychological and biological theories and corresponding treatment paradigms.

Acute Phase

Antidepressant medication is successful in 65 to 70 percent of patients in the acute care phase of major depression (Depression Guidelines Panel, 1993b). This response rate is significantly higher than the 20–30 percent (although sometimes as high as 50 percent) spontaneous remission rate or response rate to placebo. The duration and dosage of antidepressant medication are important because antidepressants have a latency period of several weeks before therapeutic effect occurs, full response may require up to six weeks of daily treatment, and there are some minimum levels considered to be adequate daily dosages (Katon et al., 1992; Depression Guidelines Panel, 1993b). Although there has been much effort to compare the efficacy of different antidepressant medications, their clinical efficacy remains largely comparable to imipramine, a commonly chosen benchmark for comparisons (Caldecott-Hazard and Schneider, 1992). Medications differ in their side effects and therefore in their appropriateness for different patients, however. Medications with sedating properties can be preferable for agitated depression, for example, but would be inappropriate for elderly patients (NIH Consensus Development Panel, 1992). Newer antidepressants, such as fluoxetine (Prozac), do not cause sedation, dry mouth, constipation, cardiac arrhythmias, and many other side effects of tricyclic antidepressants, but instead can cause agitation or anxiety, insomnia, weight loss, and nausea. Also, because some individuals respond to one type of medication but not another, successful treatment may require trying different medications.

Medications differ in their efficacy for different types of depression. MAOIs, which require a high degree of compliance in that patients must follow a reduced tyramine diet (no cheese or red wine), may be less effective than tricyclic antidepressants in endogenous forms of depression, though this conclusion is uncertain because early studies tested relatively low dosages. MAOIs are, however, very effective in depression with "atypical" symptoms, such as increased sleep and eating, marked lethargy, and interpersonal hypersensitivity (Depression Guidelines Panel, 1993b).

Minor tranquilizers or anti-anxiety medications are the most commonly used psychotropic medications. They are not approved by the Federal Drug Administration (FDA) as antidepressant medications, however, and there is little evidence for their efficacy in the acute phase, with the possible exception of alprazolam. Studies suggest that the main benefit of alprazolam may be that its effects are felt more quickly than the effects of most antidepressants (Depression Guidelines Panel, 1993b). Minor tranquilizers, including alprazolam, cause substantial withdrawal problems with long-term use (more than a few months). The Depression Guidelines Panel (1993b) does not recommend minor tranquilizers for treatment of depression unless antidepressant medications are contraindicated and only short-term treatment is feasible.

Time-limited psychotherapies (twelve to twenty sessions) are of established efficacy in the acute phase of moderate to severe depression, with a response rate of 47 to 55 percent (Depression Guidelines Panel, 1993b; Robinson, Berman, and Meimeyer, 1990). Efficacious therapies include interpersonal psychotherapy (IPT, Klerman and Weissman, 1993), individual and group forms of cognitive therapy (CT, Beck, 1962, 1967a; Covi and Lipman, 1987), and behavioral therapies including behavioral marital therapy. Brief psychodynamic psychotherapy has not been rigorously studied, but the Depression Guidelines Panel (1993b) considers it less effective than other brief therapies. Psychotherapy alone is not recommended in endogenous depression or melancholia, which responds well to antidepressant medication, nor in psychotic depression (Caldecott-Hazard and Schneider, 1992).

One might expect that the effects of antidepressant medication and psychotherapy are additive because they are such fundamentally different treatment modalities. This is an area of debate because relatively few data are available. The Depression Guidelines Panel's meta-analysis (1993b) suggested that cognitive therapy plus medication can be more effective than either treatment alone. But because other studies showed no advantage to combined treatment, the Depression Guidelines Panel recommended combined treatment when either treatment alone is only partially successful (especially in more severely ill patients and those with persistent psychosocial problems), but not for less severe major depression. Others point out that clinicians typically have not provided appropriate psychotropic medication management, a problem that should be corrected before adding another treatment modality (Caldecott-Hazard and Schneider, 1992). The World Health Organization's consensus statement (WHO, 1989) about treatment of major depression adds yet another recommendation: psychotherapy alone for mild depression, combined treatment for moderate depression, and combined treatment and / or electroconvulsive therapy (ECT) for severe depression.

Other somatic treatments have been tested in depression, but are not recommended for routine use except in tertiary care settings, and thus are not considered further in this book. They include adjunctive therapies, such as stimulants, which are sometimes used because of rapid onset of action but are problematical for long-term use; neuroleptics or antipsychotic medications, which are used as adjunctive therapy for psychotic symptoms; lithium, which can enhance treatment response to antidepressant medication; and thyroid hormone. Although the Depression Guidelines Panel (1993b) suggests that these adjunctive treatments be used only in the context of specialty referral, some of these treatments may already be used by primary care providers or through over-the-counter preparations (Caldecott-Hazard and Schneider, 1992). Other somatic therapies include ECT, which is particularly effective for severe depression with melancholic or psychotic features, persons who are not responding to other treatments or who cannot take antidepressant medications, and imminently suicidal patients. In the United States, ECT is a second-line treatment for these special circumstances, but it is still considered an important first-line treatment in other countries (WHO, 1989). Phototherapy is a new treatment with preliminary evidence for short-term efficacy (two weeks) in persons with seasonal mood disorder (a temporal relationship of symptoms over at least three years) (Oren and Rosenthal, 1992). It is viewed as a secondary treatment for this subgroup if there is a poor response to other therapies.

Continuation and Maintenance Phases

Continuation therapy is a time-limited (four-to-six-month) extension of the acute phase of treatment to prevent relapse or an exacerbation of symptoms before a complete remission occurs. Maintenance therapy is an extension to prevent recurrence, and does not have a limit on its duration. Antidepressant medications are of established efficacy in preventing recurrence (Kupfer, 1991), and such maintenance therapy is probably more effective if the full acute-phase therapeutic dosage is continued, rather than tapered to a low dosage (Frank et al., 1991; Depression Guidelines Panel, 1993b). Because not all acutely depressed persons are at risk for a recurrence, the Depression Guidelines Panel (1993b) recommends maintenance therapy only for persons with three or more prior episodes or for those with two or more episodes plus at least one other risk factor (rapid recurrence after discontinuation of medication, family history of recurrent depression, early onset of first episode, recent life-threatening episodes). The WHO consensus statement (1989) recommends maintenance therapy for persons with more than one severe episode or with several episodes in five years. Efficacy in the maintenance phase has been established for several different heterocyclic antidepressant medications, MAOIs, and fluoxetine. Antidepressant medications are also necessary in the continuation phase after a course of ECT.

Psychotherapy has not been studied much as a maintenance therapy (Frank et al., 1991, 1993), but one study found that maintenance psychotherapy (once-a-month booster sessions) delayed, but did not prevent, recurrence (Frank et al., 1990). Determining which type of treatment is effective in the maintenance phase is difficult, however, because patients might only respond to maintenance of the *same* treatment to which they responded in the acute phase (Greenhouse et al., 1991). More research on the value of psychotherapy in the maintenance phase is important because many depressed patients are women of childbearing age who cannot take antidepressant medications during pregnancy.

Effectiveness of Treatment

Although clinical trials have established whether or not a treatment works in a controlled setting, it is also important to understand the *effectiveness* of a treatment, that is, whether or not it also improves outcomes for typical patients treated in community practice settings. This is not a trivial distinction. Clinical trials provide treatments according to highly standardized or structured protocols, usually by trained study clinicians rather than usual care providers, and treatment costs are largely paid through research grants, changing provider and patient incentives. In contrast, a patient in actual practice settings may face varying costs across treatments, possibly resulting in differences in compliance (such as discontinuing an expensive drug) and, consequently, outcomes. For example, newer antidepressant medications tend to be much more expensive than older, heterocyclic medications, and patients may not be willing or able to pay these higher costs, especially if they do not feel immediate benefits. Among patients whose insurers or health care plans pay for medication, the price of medication becomes an important allocation issue. In the United States, data from the National Prescription Audit indicate that costs per prescription filled for antidepressants went up significantly faster than the number of prescriptions between 1990 and 1994. Similarly, Australia encountered a doubling in costs of antidepressant medications, despite stable prescription rates, in the four-year period after introduction of selective serotonin reuptake inhibitors (Alchin and Tranby, 1994).

In addition to different incentives, patients in efficacy studies are not representative of typical depressed patients because clinical trials tend to select "pure" clinical cases, exclude patients with comorbidities, and sample from the specialty sector in academic settings. One exception is the National Institute of Mental Health (NIMH) Collaborative Study (Elkin et al., 1989), which included outpatients. Although some of the limitations of traditional randomized clinical trials can be overcome by more generalizable "social experiment" designs, inherent theoretical and practical problems of randomized experiments will always limit their policy relevance.

How Depression Is Actually Treated

The simple existence of efficacious treatments does not mean that depressed patients receive them. Many depressed individuals do not receive health care of any kind, and when they do, the typical provider is a general medical provider, not a mental health specialist.

This raises quality concerns. General medical office visits are often very brief, and providers must deal with a range of physical and mental health concerns, though they have limited training in treating mental disorders.

More than 20 percent of adults in the general population with recent mood disorder have had no health care contact in the last six months, and only 6 percent of people with major or minor depression visit a psychiatrist. Problems of low rates of access to care are much greater in developing countries, where services and funding resources are scarce (Broadhead and Abas, 1994). Low rates of use of services could be partly due to the social stigma associated with acknowledging a mental health problem, using psychotropic medications, or receiving counseling. For example, use rates are lower among persons who think they should handle psychological problems on their own, and some women with current psychiatric disorders lower their utilization because they are concerned about the reactions of family members (Leaf et al., 1986).

Low rates of detection and appropriate treatment of depression, especially in primary care, are not unique to the United States; they have been reported in a seventeen-nation WHO study (Üstün and Sartorius, 1995), studies in the Netherlands (Van den Brink et al., 1991) and Great Britain (Blanchard, Waterreus, and Mann, 1994; Wright, 1994), and are discussed in the clinical literature of many countries (Lemelin et al., 1994).

Detection

The general medical sector is the only source of care for at least half of all depressed patients (Regier, Goldberg, and Taube, 1978; Regier et al., 1993; Wells et al., 1987), but primary care clinicians do not recognize depression in about one-half of the affected patients in this sector (Ford, 1994; Goldberg et al., 1982; Kessler, Amick, and Thompson, 1985; Kessler, Cleary, and Burke, 1985; Nielsen and Williams, 1980; Üstün and Von Korff, 1995).

Even when general medical providers recognize the presence of a mental health problem, they may be hesitant to report it in the medical record out of concerns about confidentiality and stigmatization or lower reimbursement rates for care of psychiatric, compared with physical, conditions (Rost et al., 1994). In contrast, in mental health specialty settings, where reimbursement for care is tied to mental health conditions, depression may be over diagnosed (Schulberg et al., 1985).

The clinical significance of low detection rates is not fully understood. In general, the probability of detection rises with the severity of depression, and patients most likely to benefit from treatment are also those whose depression is most likely to be detected. Given the physician's time costs of assessment, natural recovery rates, and side effects and costs of treatments, failure to detect mild depression may not be very problematical. But appropriate treatment in general medical settings cannot improve very much so long as detection remains unimproved. Low detection rates and poor documentation in the general medical sector also reduce the probability that the condition will be monitored over time. Even "watchful waiting" cannot occur in the absence of awareness of distress.

Psychotropic Medication

Appropriate antidepressant medication usage is low in primary care and even mental health specialty practices, whereas minor tranquilizer use (which is not recommended as a first-line treatment for major depressive disorder) is common (Katon et al., 1992; Olfson and Klerman, 1992, 1993). Keller et al. (1986) found that only three in ten depressed patients in general medical and mental health specialty practices used antidepressant medication, and only one in ten received effective dosages. Even among patients treated for depression, only 48 percent of psychiatric patients and 40 percent of primary care patients used an appropriate dosage of antidepressant medication, and few continued it for more than thirty days (Simon et al., 1993).[7] These low rates of treatment are surprising, considering that medications represent a "medical" model of care that should be familiar to physicians. It may be that clinicians are concerned about side effects, especially if there are comorbid illnesses and other medications.

The introduction of the newer antidepressant medications, SSRIs, is likely to result in increased rates of appropriate antidepressant treatment. According to data from the National Prescription Audit, prescriptions filled for antidepressant medications increased by 75 percent between 1990 and 1994, and costs more than doubled. Prescriptions for older antidepressant medications (tricyclics) remained fairly constant, although their market share fell as a result of a three-fold increase in the number of prescriptions for SSRIs such as fluoxetine. This increase in sales could not be explained by population growth, and therefore represents higher prescription rates per capita. Antidepressant medications are prescribed for problems other than depression (for example, newer antidepressants are used to treat obsessive-compulsive disorders), and the number of prescriptions filled does not completely correspond to medication usage, which is affected by compliance. As a result, we cannot calculate from these trends how much the rates of antidepressant medication use have changed among depressed patients. The prevalence of newer antidepressants can lead to higher effective use rates if prescribed for depression, as depressed patients receiving them are more likely than patients receiving older antidepressants to continue their medication for more than thirty days and to receive an appropriate dosage.

Psychotherapy

Psychotherapy is more difficult than psychotropic medications to evaluate because it is not the same in typical health care settings as it is in clinical trials, where specific manualized protocols such as cognitive or interpersonal psychotherapy predominate. There are no professional standards in any provider sector that limit counseling to psychotherapies of known efficacy, and monitoring sessions to assure compliance would be very difficult and costly. General medical providers appear to counsel depressed patients in brief, problem-oriented encounters that include elements of psychotherapy, but primarily provide advice and reassurance (Magruder-Habib et al., 1989; Olfson and Pincus, 1994b; Orleans et al., 1985; Ormel et al., 1991; Radecki and Mendenhall, 1986). Although this is not a formal psychotherapy of proven efficacy, it is the most common form of counseling for depressed patients. Some have argued that all therapeutic encounters rely on common elements such as empathy, suggesting that both formal psychotherapies and more informal medical counseling may have therapeutic value (Frank, 1961). Thus, developing methods of defining and describing counseling for depression as typically practiced and measuring its effectiveness are among the field's unresolved research challenges.

The problem of evaluating counseling in usual care settings is not unique to depression, but applies also to preventive counseling regarding smoking and exercise (Wells et al., 1984a) or adherence with treatment. Clinicians consider counseling to be important, and the AHCPR guidelines for treating major depression recommend patient and family counseling regarding treatment compliance (Depression Guidelines Panel, 1993b).

Because of these measurement problems, studies usually rely on clinician or client reports of counseling without detailed process descriptions (Magruder-Habib et al., 1989; Olfson and Pincus, 1994a, b), which may overestimate the use of efficacious psychotherapy. Nevertheless, few depressed patients in general medical practices appear to receive formal psychotherapy (Hankin and Oktay, 1979; Johnson, 1973; Schurman, Mitchell, and Kramer, 1985; Wells et al., 1987). Even among patients diagnosed by their general medical provider as depressed, only a third receive psychotherapy or counseling, whereas almost all detected patients in psychiatry do (Olfson and Pincus, 1994a, b).

Improving the Quality of Depression Care

Prior studies of quality improvement have focused on the feasibility of changing treatment. Most studies evaluated strategies to improve clinician detection of depression through providing feedback on symptoms or diagnosis, sometimes coupled with recommendations for treatment. These studies found mixed and often discouraging results, in terms of improvements in either process or outcomes of care (Attkisson and Zich, 1990; Badger and Rand, 1988; Gerber et al., 1989; German et al., 1987; Hoeper et al., 1984; Linn and Yager, 1982; Magruder-Habib et al., 1990; Shapiro et al., 1987), although some studies using more comprehensive and intensive strategies, such as a coordinated primary care and mental health specialty effort to provide appropriate care for depression, were more successful (Brody et al., 1990; Katon et al., 1995). Problems in demonstrating effectiveness or cost-effectiveness of quality improvement are not unique to care of depression, however, and reflect both the early stage of development of this field and the complexity of changing clinician behavior.

Treatment decisions are influenced by data on efficacy, costs, and side effects of treatments. Most clinicians would consider prevailing treatment rates to be unacceptably low, but are the costs of higher-quality care worth it from the perspective of benefits to plans, employers, patients, and society? This brings us to the social role of depression, for without data on the costs and benefits for different participants groups (patients, providers, employers, insurers), it may not be possible to determine the main obstacles to efficient care and achievement of lasting changes.

Chapter Three

The Social Role of Depression and Health Care Policy

A policy perspective considers how depression and its treatment affect society and, by calculating the social costs of a disease, how depression compares with other conditions. Social costs can be high if a health condition is common and substantially affects people's functioning and well-being, even if the condition does not have dramatic mortality rates or require costly treatments.

If the distribution of social costs were immutable, studying them would be of little policy interest. Social costs can be influenced by health care policy, however. For example, raising the incentives for aggressively treating one condition through generous reimbursement rates for providers increases its direct treatment costs, but may reduce indirect social costs through the reduced morbidity and mortality that result from more appropriate care.

In the United States, recent policy debates have focused on two dimensions of health care delivery that are likely to affect treatment rates: the role of payment systems and the role of specialty care. In this chapter we review the connection between these policy choices and care for depression, although little is known about how payment systems or provider specialty affects patient outcomes, cost-effectiveness, or social costs.

Societal Impact of Depression

How Common Is Depression?

Estimates of the prevalence of depression are important for planning prevention, access to care, or treatment programs, and to anticipate program costs. Current estimates vary depending on definitions, assessment methods, and sample. The most important distinction is between community and patient samples.

Community Prevalence

Major depressive and dysthymic disorders are among the most common psychiatric disorders worldwide, and may even be as common as many typical medical problems. The two main U.S. studies of the prevalence of depression are the National Institute of Mental Health Epidemiologic Catchment Area (ECA) Program and the National Comorbidity Study (NCS).[1] The latest analysis of the ECA data estimated that major depressive disorder has a one-year prevalence of 5 percent, meaning that one in twenty people experiences major depression in any year; the one-year prevalence estimate of dysthymic disorder was 5.4 percent (Regier et al., 1993). This makes major depressive and dysthymic disorders the third and fourth most common specific psychiatric disorders, after phobia (11 percent) and alcohol-use disorder (7 percent). The NCS estimates of one-year prevalence were even higher for major depression (10.3 percent), but lower for dysthymic disorder (2.5 percent) (Blazer et al., 1994; Kessler et al., 1994).[2]

Lifetime prevalence rates from community surveys are more suspect than current prevalence rates, because they are more subject to recall bias. In the NCS, lifetime prevalence of major depressive disorder was 17.1 percent; lifetime prevalence of dysthymic disorder was 6.4 percent (Blazer et al., 1994; Kessler et al., 1994).

Studies in other nations using methods similar to the ECA's report lifetime rates of major depression that vary from a low of 0.9–1.7 percent in Taiwan to a high of 8.6 percent in Edmonton, Canada (Spaner, Bland, and Newman, 1994; Weissman and Klerman, 1992). The Depression Guidelines Panel (1993a) suggested that 2–3 percent of men and 4–9 percent of women have major depressive disorder in a year, with lifetime risk of 7–12 percent for men and 20–25 percent for women, although these lifetime risk numbers seem to be too high. Lifetime rates for women in studies (excluding Asian countries) using either the DIS (DSM-III) or Present State Examination (ICD-9) are typically in the 4–16 percent (but mostly 4–8 percent) range for major depression, and in the 4–8 percent range for dysthymia (Smith and Weissman, 1992).

The prevalence of major depressive disorder appears to be increasing over time and by birth cohort, according to findings from the ECA and several other countries (Klerman and Weissman, 1989). Despite variations by site, possibly attributable to local political events or other environmental factors (Cross-National Collaborative Group, 1992), the time trend in the rate of increase is too great to be explained by changes in the gene pool. Some believe that methods effects (reporting biases) contribute to the higher rates in younger cohorts (Simon and Von Korff, 1992), but others have suggested that this may be an effect of economic conditions such as recessions (Madianos and Stefanis, 1992).

Prevalence among Patients

The prevalence of clinically meaningful depressive symptoms is generally in the 15–30 percent range among primary care patients, but rates ranging from 6 to 94 percent have been published (Zung et al., 1993). The prevalence in U.S. primary care samples of major depressive disorder varies from about 5 percent to 9 percent across studies; rates for dysthymic disorder range between 2 percent and 4 percent; minor depression between 3 percent and 5 percent; and intermittent depression rates are around 5 percent (Katon and Schulberg, 1992; Katon and Sullivan, 1990; Miranda, Hohmann, and Attkisson, 1994; Von Korff et al., 1987). Rosenblatt et al. (1983) found that anxiety and depression was the fifth most common diagnosis group in outpatient ambulatory practices, but there remains little data on how depression compares with other common physical health conditions. The seventeen-nation World Health Organization Study found an average prevalence rate of 10 percent for major depressive disorder in primary care, and a range from 3 percent in Nagasaki to 30 percent in Santiago (Goldberg and Lecrubier, 1995). Variations in rates among treated samples can result from differences in base disorder rates for populations eligible to use services, methods effects such as cultural differences in interpretation of symptoms, or differences in help-seeking patterns.

In mental health specialty settings, depression is much more prevalent, but there have been fewer representative studies. Mezzich, Coffman, and Goodpastor (1982) reported that depression accounts for at least 20 percent of outpatient mental health specialty patients.[3] Overall, there have been no data on patients of clinicians in solo practices or for comparisons across different delivery and practice settings. The MOS filled this gap, comparing the prevalence of depression with some common physical problems, and the results are presented in Chapter 6.

Risk Factors for Depression

Some groups are at higher risk for depression than others, and this information can be useful in targeting them for specific interventions or services. Women, for example, are about twice as likely as men to be depressed, although this discrepancy may be partly explained by differences in the way men and women respond to questions about symptoms (Wilhelm and Parker, 1994).

African Americans are less likely than Hispanics or whites (who have similar rates) to suffer from major depression, but are more likely to have other psychiatric comorbidities when depressed (Blazer et al., 1994). Little is known about prevalence of depression among Asian Americans, although Chinese in Taiwan have very low rates of depressive disorders, and Koreans in Seoul have rates at the lower range for the ECA communities (Weissman and Klerman, 1992).

Young adults and persons with less education have higher rates of major depressive disorder, and more psychiatric comorbidity when depressed. In the United States, there are no regional or urban / rural differences after controlling for economic or sociodemographic differences (Kessler et al., 1994).

In Finland, depression increases in prevalence for women through middle age and then declines (Lehtinen and Joukamaa, 1994), although older Finnish adults have a high prevalence of dysthymic disorder—17 percent in men and 23 percent in women (Kivela and Pahkala, 1989).

Aside from demographic factors, the main risk factors for major depressive disorder include a family history of depression and alcoholism, a prior personal history of depression, and possibly a history of marital separation or divorce (Bromet et al., 1990). In a sample of an urban African American community, the strongest risk factors for major depressive disorder besides age were poor physical health and a high level of stressful life events; this study was unusual, however, in that it did not find a significant difference between men and women (Brown et al., 1995).

In treated samples, these risk factors for depression may be enhanced or masked by factors affecting help-seeking behavior. For example, women are more likely than men to use general and mental health services, but among users of mental health services, men are relatively more likely to seek specialty care (which could mask some of the sex differences in depression risk in that sector) (Leaf et al., 1985). Patients receiving mental health services from general medical providers are on average older, more physically ill, and have less education than users of mental health specialty services (Wells et al., 1987). Although the WHO seventeen-nation study found that there was great variability across sites in risk factors for major depressive disorder among primary care attenders, females and those with less education were more likely to be depressed (Goldberg and Lecrubier, 1995).

Social Costs of Depression

Indirect social costs are the costs to society of an illness or its treatment other than direct treatment costs. They include loss of work and productivity (for example, housework) resulting from sickness, and time costs related to obtaining care.

Economic studies have tried to determine the relative contribution of mortality, morbidity, and treatment costs to social losses for a given clinical condition and across conditions. The most recent study estimates the annual social costs of affective disorders to be around $44 billion, an amount that exceeds the social costs of coronary heart disease or arthritis (Greenberg et al., 1993). This study and earlier research (Kind and Sorensen, 1993; Dorothy Rice et al., 1990; Stoudemire et al., 1986) confirm the substantial indirect (non–health care) costs of affective disorders caused by morbidity. In fact, indirect costs, which include reduced productivity of the depressed person and the burdens of family members who spend time caring for a sick relative, far exceed direct treatment costs. Morbidity costs attributable to reduced productivity in depression ($24 billion in 1990) account for more than half the total social costs and are twice as high as the direct treatment costs ($12 billion). Thus, unlike other medical conditions, depression is significant for its high associated morbidity, not for its high direct treatment costs or mortality. Indeed, morbidity is the key policy outcome for evaluating care of depression.

In contrast, suicide is the most important clinical concern. Even though suicide accounts for many deaths among young adults in the United States (Klerman, 1987) and was the seventh leading cause of death in the United States overall between 1970 and 1992 (U.S. Bureau of the Census, 1994), cardiovascular diseases, cancer, chronic lung diseases and pneumonia, and even accidents cause many more deaths. For example, in 1991, suicide accounted for 12 deaths per 100,000 persons, whereas cardiovascular diseases accounted for 362 deaths per 100,000, and accidents for 36 deaths per 100,000. Individuals with chronic medical conditions such as heart disease are on average much older than depressed persons, but even when adjusting for age differences, heart disease and cancer account for ten to fifteen times as many deaths as suicide. Thus, if mortality were the only contributor to social costs, depression would be much less of a burden on society than it is when morbidity is considered.

Although the overall conclusions of cost-of-illness studies are likely to remain valid, there are still large substantive and methodological gaps. For example, consider the studies of workplace incapacitation caused by depression. This impact can be estimated through the human capital framework, under which one would examine market wages as a function of health status, including level of depression. In a competitive economy, market wages would reflect the marginal contribution a person makes to society. But in order to estimate an income equation in an appropriate human capital framework, much more information is needed than income and mental health status, which is all that has been available. In the absence of such data, estimates are likely to be influenced by many other confounding factors and selection biases. For example, depression appears to be positively correlated with higher socioeconomic status. Consequently, it is not surprising that major depression and dysthymia are associated at a point in time with greater earnings for all age groups and for both males and females in community samples (Rice and Miller, 1993, table 3), but this is only a consequence of data limitations. Such problems severely handicap the validity of cost-of-illness studies: Rice and Miller (1993), for example, assumed that depression had no effect on income; and Greenberg et al. (1993) made the arbitrary assumption that depression decreases an individual's productivity at work by 20 percent, similar to the effect of any mental illness on earnings (Frank and Gertler, 1991).

Unfortunately, our knowledge about the relationship between depression, job changes, labor force participation, and wealth accumulation remains quite limited.[4] Labor economics provides the necessary conceptual and analytical tools, but new data bases that include both health and economic information are necessary. The MOS did not obtain economic data, and we cannot address the issue of indirect costs of depression or consequences of treatment for indirect costs, except for the change in income associated with changes in functioning limitations.

Health Care Policy and Care of Depression

In some countries, health care is publicly provided, and the government plays a direct role in determining the type and quality of services. In many other countries, including the United States, health care is largely private and indirectly influenced by governmental policies regulating reimbursement for publicly funded patients (Medicare and Medicaid), licensing of providers, and insurance. In the United States, the role of publicly provided health care (for example, state hospitals for the severely mentally ill) is relatively small, and the private sector supports a diverse market with competing financing and delivery systems. This competition has given rise to managed care, cost-containment strategies, and prepaid (PP) care—developments that are closely watched in other countries, including France, that try to control costs through increased management of services within the context of a pluralistic, mixed private-public system (Bach, 1994; Petchey, 1987). Some former socialist countries have recently converted to a private delivery system, often implementing fee-for-service (FFS) reimbursement mechanisms (Massaro, Nemec, and Kalman, 1994); as their systems evolve, they may want to rely on experience gained in the United States.

In this book, we focus on two central dimensions of current policy debates in the United States: the role of financing and reimbursement strategies in private care and the role of specialty care. We analyze these issues from a quality-of-care and cost-effectiveness perspective, which is relevant for most wealthy countries. An analysis appropriate to developing countries, many of which are rethinking the financing and organization of their health care systems (World Bank, 1987, 1993), might instead study how changes in financing affect both the redistribution of resources toward poorer segments of the population and the role of private markets (Gertler and Sturm, forthcoming).

Financing

The two main private-sector financing systems differ in their incentives for health care utilization: PP arrangements encourage providers (the supply side of health care utilization) to reduce costs, because providers do not receive additional reimbursement for any particular service; FFS plans encourage the enrollee or patient (the demand side) to lower utilization through copayments (Ellis and McGuire, 1993; McGuire, 1993). Both financing types also employ nonprice mechanisms, such as office hours and waiting times, and managed-care strategies, such as utilization review and gatekeeping, to limit utilization and control access to specialists or procedures. Managed care is a more recent trend among FFS arrangements, however, whereas it was always a central element of PP care.

Within each financing system there are different delivery organizations, and the MOS was the first study to sample a wide variety of organizations providing PP and FFS care. The traditional form of PP care is the group-practice style HMOs, which have been the focus of most studies of PP care. New forms of PP care that have grown rapidly in recent years include independent practice associations (IPAs) of individual providers, multispecialty group practice IPAs, multiple-specialty group practices that offer a mixture of PP and FFS arrangements on a per-patient basis, and point-of-service plans that offer different reimbursement rates on a visit basis depending on the location of use (Hoy, Curtis, and Rice, 1991; Thomas Rice et al., 1990). In FFS care, plans differ in covered benefits and reimbursement generosity levels (copayments and coinsurance, deductibles), and vary in use of managed-care strategies, such as utilization review or clinical practice guidelines.

Some other changes are more recent and have occurred since the MOS (Wells, Astrachan, Tischler, and Ünützer, 1995). The most important is the growth of so-called carve-out or managed behavioral health care companies, which specialize in the management of care for mental disorders and substance abuse. Point-of-service plans and the diffusion of managed care under FFS arrangements, such as preferred provider organizations (PPOs), are also relatively new and largely replace unmanaged FFS plans.

The first research on the role of financing studied the effects of price on demand for mental health services and health outcomes in FFS plans, which dominated the market prior to the 1990s. Reducing the patient's price for services (that is, reduced copayments) increases utilization; moreover, the price response for mental health care may be stronger than the price response for medical care (Frank and McGuire, 1986; Keeler et al., 1988). In terms of health outcomes, cost-sharing (higher prices) may have a negative effect for sicker and poorer individuals, but there is no average effect across plans (Wells, Manning, and Valdez, 1989). Nevertheless, this raises the question of whether disadvantaged individuals are at particular risk for adverse outcomes under cost-containment strategies that rely on patient cost-sharing.

Utilization comparisons of FFS plans and well-established HMOs found that HMO patients were as likely as patients in FFS plans to have any contact with a mental health specialist in a year, but more likely to receive mental health care in the general medical sector and have fewer mental health specialty visits (Diehr, Williams, and Martin, 1985; Wells, Manning, and Benjamin, 1986). A utilization difference even existed among patients receiving mental health specialty procedures (such as psychological assessment or psychotherapy), because HMOs also relied on less expensive forms of mental health care (nonphysicians, group therapy) for those patients (Wells, Manning, and Benjamin, 1986). This commonly found result is unlikely to be caused by selection biases in observational studies, as several studies found no differences in general or mental health status between HMOs or FFS plans (Diehr, Williams, and Martin, 1985; Diehr et al., 1984; Norquist and Wells, 1991). In the Health Insurance Experiment, health outcomes were similar in the HMO studied and FFS plans (Wells, Manning, and Valdez, 1990). One study of capitated versus FFS coverage for Medicaid patients with severe mental illness found, however, that psychopathology and functioning were worse for schizophrenic patients in the capitated system (Lurie et al., 1992), although this result was not robust and was not observed for more specific outcomes.

Specialty

Specialty mix is a main determinant of overall health care costs and possibly health outcomes, an issue that has gained visibility with trends to increase the proportion of physicians in primary care disciplines and to rely on primary care gatekeepers for controlling access to mental health specialists. Yet there has been almost no research on the impact of gatekeeper systems or shifting specialty mix on costs, quality, or outcomes of mental health care.

Patients receiving their mental health care only in the general medical sector tend to have only a few mental health visits a year, whereas patients of mental health specialists average ten or more visits annually (Wells et al., 1987). For persons with affective disorder in the ECA, the average number of mental health specialty visits was seventeen, and the average number of general medical visits was five (Narrow et al., 1993).

The only randomized trial assigned 121 depressed general medical patients in Great Britain to usual care by the general practitioner, antidepressant medication by a psychiatrist, cognitive therapy by a psychologist, or counseling and case work by a social worker. Outcomes were not consistently different, but costs were twice as high under specialty care, and the authors concluded that mental health specialty care was not cost-effective in outpatient care for acute depression (Scott and Freeman, 1992). The randomized design of this study avoided bias in selection that could result in systematic patient health differences across sector, but the small sample size made it impossible to detect small but clinically meaningful outcome differences.[5] We will revisit the cost-effectiveness of care by different specialists in Chapter 10, using the nonexperimental MOS design on a larger sample of severely depressed patients.

Chapter Four

Evaluating Health Care Systems

The quality of evaluation studies depends on how well the design and analytic framework relate to the research questions. Following a cookbook formula will rarely yield a cost-effective study, and seemingly minor differences in design, instruments, and analytic methods can render contradictory conclusions. Such methodological issues seldom get the attention they deserve because methodological details are often deleted or at least relegated to the small print in clinical and health services research publications. Although the absence of appropriate measures and data can render even the most elegant analysis useless, many seem to believe that an evaluation requires only the use of an appropriate questionnaire, without realizing the dominating role of analytic methods.

The best way to illustrate design and analytic decision problems is to present a concrete example, which we do in the context of the MOS. The MOS research questions ranged from classical epidemiologic questions to clinical problems and even economic evaluations:

1. How prevalent is depression in typical general medical practices and mental health specialty practices, and how does it compare with medical conditions?
2. How limited are depressed patients in their daily functioning and well-being, and how do they compare with patients with medical conditions?
3. How does treatment differ by specialty and payment system?
4. How do outcomes differ by specialty and payment system?
5. How can care for depression become more cost-effective?

There is some tension among these research questions, and the MOS needed a design that addressed all of them within a limited budget, a problem that arises in all evaluations. The MOS approach reflects an attempt to bridge clinical treatment and health services research needs, and this integration led to insights that would not have been possible without compromising between different research approaches. Nevertheless, not all areas could be addressed equally well: epidemiologic research (question 1) and economics (question 5) had a lower priority than studying the impact of depression on individuals (question 2), evaluating the appropriateness of care as usual (question 3), and comparing health outcomes across practice settings (question 4).

In this chapter we discuss general design issues, then describe the measurement framework for the MOS, and finally provide an overview of the MOS design.

Observational and Experimental Designs

Randomized experimental designs are often considered inherently superior to observational approaches, a clinical research paradigm that is often advocated for social policy evaluations. The advantages of an experimental design are balanced by a similar number of disadvantages, however. As experience in other areas, such as job training programs or unemployment compensation schemes, shows, social experiments have not always provided better answers to policy questions (Heckman and Smith, 1995).

Whether experimental or observational, most evaluations try to answer a question like the following: What would outcomes have been if a group of people had received a different treatment than they actually did? This question cannot be answered directly, because the same individual outcomes with and without treatment are not observable, and both experimental and observational approaches need to construct this counterfactual scenario. Experiments randomly assign individuals to different treatments to guarantee that the groups compared are similar, whereas the simplest observational approaches rely only on statistical methods to assure that the groups compared are similar. Natural experiments or quasi-experiments (Cook and Campbell, 1979; Cook and Shadish, 1994; Meyer, 1995) are observational studies that incorporate into the design exogenous variations, such as changes in laws or regulations, to strengthen the similarity of compared groups in observational studies.

Threats to the validity of evaluation results are commonly grouped into external and internal threats (Campbell, 1957; Cook and Campbell, 1979). External validity means that the results can be generalized, and it is endangered if the sample or the practice settings are not representative. This is where observational designs can have a significant advantage over experimental designs: individuals, providers, or practices are more likely to participate in studies that do not require them to change their activities, reducing selective enrollment biases. Experimental studies need to provide significantly larger bonuses to achieve similar participation rates, which substantially affect the size of the sample for a given research budget.

The cheaper design and reduced burden on participants of observational studies also allow a wider range of participants and samples, an essential element in studying the effectiveness of care. In an observational study, many of the exclusion criteria necessary in clinical trials no longer apply, making patient participants much more representative of typical depressed patients. An observational study also requires no skills to follow research protocols from practices, reducing the bias toward well-established or academic settings.

To obtain generalizable results on the effectiveness of care, one also needs to study care as usual in typical practice settings. This is where experimental designs fail because the necessary constraints of randomization alter the functioning of the health care delivery system. For example, one could assign depressed patients to PP or FFS care (or different types of providers), but this would disrupt existing patient-provider relationships. Such a study would no longer provide externally valid results on how financing systems or specialty sectors differ in their care as usual.

The internal validity of a study is threatened if differences in the dependent variable are caused by something other than differences in the explanatory variables, such as unmeasured variables, simultaneity between dependent and explanatory variables (the dependent variable causally predicts the value of some explanatory variable), misspecified statistical models, differential attrition between comparison groups, or other selection effects. These problems are common in both experimental designs and observational studies. Clinical studies often remove from a trial individuals who become too sick, and patients' participation rates differ among the comparison groups according to the treatment offered in nonblind studies (which all social experiments are). In the Health Insurance Experiment, refusal rates in the free plan were a third of those in the high coinsurance plan, and attrition rates among families who initially accepted the plans were also lower in the free plan—despite carefully designed side payments that made the plans similarly attractive financially (Newhouse et al., 1993). These problems can render simple statistical comparisons invalid, even in experimental studies.

The problem of selection bias is much more important in nonexperimental designs, however, where it may be the single most important concern. Because policy results are always interpreted causally—if not by the scientific community then certainly by the press and decision-makers—it is inappropriate to rely on simple statistics with a disclaimer that results should only be interpreted descriptively, instead of explicitly addressing the problem of selection biases.

Selection Biases

The difference in outcomes between comparison groups includes the treatment effect and the selection effect that are consequences of sorting on unmeasured characteristics. Selection bias is generally a consequence of missing variables: if the characteristics of comparison groups were comprehensively measured, one could select perfect comparison groups or control for these effects statistically. A particularly important variable is health status, as sicker patients typically have a poorer prognosis than healthier patients, regardless of treatment effects. As a result, a naive direct outcome comparison of two different sectors that ignores sickness differences is biased against the one starting with initially sicker patients. For example, patients of the MOS psychiatrists experienced on average ten depressive symptoms in the second year of the MOS, whereas patients of the MOS general medical providers experienced six symptoms. This clearly means not that psychiatrists achieve worse outcomes than general medical clinicians, but that there are differences in casemix.

By contrast, more depressed patients generally improve more than less depressed individuals (the "regression to the mean" phenomenon), even if they remain sicker. A similarly misleading analysis focusing on changes in health status is therefore biased against the sector starting with initially less sick patients. Compared with year one, patients of psychiatrists have two fewer depressive symptoms in year two, whereas patients of general medical providers improve only half as much.

The same contradictory results can appear in a naive comparison of treated and untreated patients because sickness is a predictor of treatment. Regressing mental health status (measured by the five-item mental health inventory) at year one on effective antidepressant medication suggests a highly significant negative effect ($p < 0.01$) of antidepressant medication on mental health. Analyzing the change in mental health (year one minus baseline) gives the opposite results—that antidepressant medications improve mental health.

Despite this sensitivity to changes in the statistical analysis, we are not pessimistic about the value of observational studies. The sensitivity by itself is not a cause of concern because research that fails to account for selection effects is flawed and few people would be surprised to learn that this results in wrong conclusions. But the sensitivity does reveal a need to improve the methodological standards in published research. As these examples show, it may not be too difficult to find a way to confirm a desirable hypothesis or refute an undesirable one. Under these circumstances, how credible are claims of significant relationships in the absence of comprehensive case-mix adjustments, appropriate statistical models, and sensitivity analyses?

Two complementary approaches have been explored in other research fields that traditionally had to rely on observational data. Econometrics has a long tradition of statistical methods for nonexperimental data, focusing on selection models and specification tests to identify incorrect assumptions and false models (Heckman, 1990; Heckman and Hotz, 1989).[1] Some researchers have suggested that selection models are based on different assumptions and do not necessarily replicate experimental findings (LaLonde, 1986), and recent developments have addressed some of these concerns (Heckman and Smith, 1995). A traditional economic technique that has recently been explored in health is instrumental variable estimation (McClellan, 1995; McClellan, McNeil, and Newhouse, 1994).[2] Instrumental variable estimation tries to mimic the effect of random assignment in experiments by breaking the correlation between unobserved factors and explanatory variables. For outcome evaluations, for example, instrumental variable estimation uses observable factors (instruments) that influence treatment but do not directly affect patient outcomes. Finding instrumental variables is not a trivial design issue, however, and a poor choice can exacerbate the existing problems (Bound, Jaeger, and Baker, 1995). In addition, instrumental variable methods have lower statistical power, which in the design of the study must be compensated with increased sample sizes.

Another way to avoid the misleading conclusions that can result from a poorly chosen model is to study the sensitivity of results and conclusions to different modeling assumptions (Leamer, 1983, 1985), which was the primary approach in the MOS. For example, a simple sensitivity analysis would compare the qualitative findings of end-status (that is, end of follow-up period) and change analyses (endpoint minus baseline) to determine the effect of selection biases. But there is no substitute for detailed health status measures, and we found that many qualitative results only became robust when comprehensive baseline health status measures were included in the analysis.[3] Because the central potential source of selection bias was related to health status in the MOS, the MOS paid particular attention to health status and case-mix measurement. For other evaluations, important selection biases could result from non-health dimensions.[4]

Other Design Issues

Tracer Condition Approach

General population or patient samples deal with a broad range of health problems, whereas a tracer condition approach samples patients with specific health conditions. A tracer condition approach becomes particularly useful for clinically detailed health outcomes or quality-of-care comparisons because general samples of the same size do not yield enough patients with the same conditions to allow meaningful comparisons across systems of care or health conditions.

Good tracer conditions are health conditions whose treatment or prevention implications are well understood.[5] With a tracer approach, evaluations can chart the effectiveness of different components of a health care delivery system by examining whether care is adequate. Different conditions place different demands on various aspects of the health care delivery system, such as a delivery system's capacity to provide preventive care, its ability to provide acute (emergency) care, or its propensity to provide chronic (rehabilitation) care.

A depression tracer evaluates a delivery system's ability to identify and manage a seriously ill group in both an acute and a maintenance phase (for example, ongoing antidepressant medication to prevent or delay recurrence of major depression). This is a more demanding test of a delivery system than a pregnancy-care tracer, for example, which evaluates how well a system manages relatively healthy women over a clearly defined period. To maximize the variation of treatments, it is particularly useful to identify patients with a tracer condition independent from the treating provider.

Different types of depression vary in their properties as tracer conditions. The MOS included three: major depressive disorder, dysthymic disorder, and subthreshold depression. Major depressive disorder is an excellent tracer condition because there is little disagreement about its definition, there are many alternative efficacious treatments available, and there is considerable variation in treatments across providers. Dysthymic disorder may also be a good tracer condition, but there is less evidence on the efficacy of treatment. Subthreshold depression is probably the weakest tracer because it represents a heterogeneous set of conditions and there is little evidence on the efficacy of treatment.

Study Duration

Clinical studies are typically very short, with follow-up periods measured in weeks or months, whereas longitudinal economic or social science studies are generally long, with follow-up surveys taking place once a year or every other year. These time dimensions are driven by the study questions: economic and social phenomena, such as job changes or educational achievement, change slowly; clinical symptoms change quickly. Economic studies are willing to forgo clinical detail to study long-term effects on wealth and labor market status over many years. Drug trials in turn give up the ability to measure life-cycle effects in favor of demonstrating short-term efficacy. The MOS compromised between these two approaches by repeating interviews at six-month intervals to capture some quickly changing health effects, but continued this over two years (with an additional survey after four years) to address long-term effects. This compromise allows us to examine how an individual's functioning and well-being are affected by a serious acute condition such as major depression compared with a chronic condition such as dysthymia. A short-term (clinical) study would be biased against conditions with less immediate impact, even if they led to greater impairment over time, whereas a long-term economic or social science study could miss the dramatic short-term effects of an acute illness.

Enrollee Versus Patient Samples

The MOS focused on a patient rather than an enrollee sample, which would include individuals not using services. A patient sample provides a better contrast for quality-of-care comparisons across systems of care because systems have less control over nonusers.

Enrollee samples can be more generalizable, however, because the reference population is easily defined, whereas patients can be in and out of treatment and a reference patient panel can be hard to define. Some issues, such as access to care, require an enrollee sample; others, such as detection of a specific condition, require a patient sample. The MOS depression study has some features of an access study in that patients were included in the depression study regardless of whether or not they explicitly sought care for depression.

Among patient sample designs, one can select all patients, new patients, or established patients. The MOS required an ongoing care relationship and did not include patients receiving only a consultation from a MOS clinician. This is a cost-effective sampling design because only a minority of *new* patients return to the same provider. In addition, this strategy resulted in a sample more likely to be exposed over time to the practice style of the participating clinician, which increases the value of the physician measures. The disadvantage of sampling ongoing care patients is that they may have already received some acute-phase care, which could underestimate treatment benefits.

Variety of Practice Settings and Sample Sizes

The question of how many different practices to include and how many types of delivery systems to study is mainly a research cost and feasibility issue, as it is important to ensure that each type contributes enough patients for a meaningful comparison. Many studies can only consider two or three specific settings for budgetary reasons, such as patients from one HMO and from one FFS plan. To improve the generalizability and representativeness, however, one would do better to sample from different practices or plans of the same type in different areas, even if the number of patients is the same. This may preclude an analysis of a particular practice, which would be a problem if the goal is to rate a particular practice. If one is interested in systematic differences across groups of similar types of practices or plans, however, it is advantageous to include a large number of practices and plans, as the MOS did. Many practices contributed fewer than ten depressed patients, and only the HMOs in the MOS contributed enough patients to test for individual practice effects. Because no individual practice can dominate the results, the MOS conclusions about types of delivery system are much more generalizable than if they were based on two or three practices, even with the same patient sample size.

The number of comparison groups (that is, delivery systems in the MOS) to include depends on the desired precision of results, which in turn is influenced by the variables measured and the sample size for each group. More observations per group quickly increase precision, but some variables require many more observations than others to obtain similarly confident statistical conclusions. Thus the important design issue of how many groups to compare requires consideration of research questions and measures simultaneously.

Well-Established Practice Settings

The MOS focused on well-established practice settings with clinicians who were board-certified, board-eligible, or licensed for independent clinical practice, and who had practiced in these settings for several years. This simplified the organization of the project (contacting providers and maintaining continuity over the course of the study) and reduced heterogeneity at the practice and provider level, which improves statistical precision. But this approach may result in overestimation of the quality of care relative to that provided in all practice settings, reducing the external validity of the study, although the bias is in a known direction. This seems a relatively minor problem compared with the need for voluntary cooperation from practices in all studies, which is likely to be a larger threat to generalizability.

Different health care settings may draw providers and patients from different geographic areas, creating another possibility for non-comparable provider or patient groups. The MOS therefore tried to match groups of providers in different practice settings within the same geographic area.

Design Effects

The MOS sampled many patients from the same provider and clinic and, in the longitudinal analysis, collected repeated observations on the same patient. As a consequence, observations are unlikely to be independent (owing to unobserved patient, physician, or clinic characteristics), and this biases standard errors and incorrect inferences. There are two general approaches: the first is a simple nonparametric correction that is appropriate in many circumstances; the second relies on more detailed modeling of the assumed correlations.[6] The MOS mainly used the nonparametric approach, although this approach does not take full advantage of the panel characteristics of the data.

Participation Incentives

The Health Insurance Experiment provided very strong financial incentives to participate, whereas the MOS provided very little ($5 per questionnaire). Clearly, the need to provide incentives is much more urgent in experimental designs that force people to change their usual activities than in observational studies that only require responding to questionnaires or interviews. But relatively minor increases in incentives in observational studies could have a dramatic impact on participation rates without being a major burden on total study costs. Overall, the MOS response rates among depressed patients were acceptable, but not very good (around 70 percent for self-reported questionnaires and 75 percent for telephone interviews). This nonresponse is sufficiently high to raise concerns about attrition and response biases, especially as more depressed patients were less likely to return questionnaires. Whereas there are many statistical methods to control biases (weighting observations, using covariates as controls in regression analysis, selection models), there is no perfect substitute for more complete data that can be obtained with strong patient incentives and intensive follow-up of nonrespondents.

MOS Depression Measurement Framework

An analysis can only be as good as the data it uses. Developing a strong data base requires a measurement framework based on theories that link the project's key variables to the key inputs and outputs of care. Our measurement framework of care for depressed patients (whether or not they explicitly seek care for depression and whether or not they or their providers recognize the depression) builds on Donabedian's (1988) three-part quality-of-care model: structure of health care delivery systems, clinical processes of care, and outcomes. Quality of care refers to aspects of process of care that affect patient outcomes, independent of other factors (such as severity of illness) affecting these outcomes.

The traditional process-of-care components of quality of care are treatments that are efficacious and should be used—or treatments that are not efficacious and should be avoided. We add processes of care that are of clinical interest or affect costs of care, even when their association with health outcomes is not established, such as clinicians' usual counseling and interpersonal style of care, use of mental health services, and continuity of care. Other factors influence health outcomes only indirectly through quality of care, such as characteristics of health care delivery systems, providers, and patients (see Figure 4.1).

Cost-effectiveness studies that address clinical and economic issues simultaneously provide the highest contribution to the development of policy priorities. The MOS emphasized health outcomes, which involve more complex measurement issues than treatment costs. In this book, therefore, we discuss only assessment of health status and quality of care, not cost or utilization, even though we analyze the cost-effectiveness of quality improvement and one managed-care strategy (Chapter 9).

Structure of the Health Care Delivery System

In organizing a study like the MOS, to contrast complex health care delivery systems one can either model individual components of or-

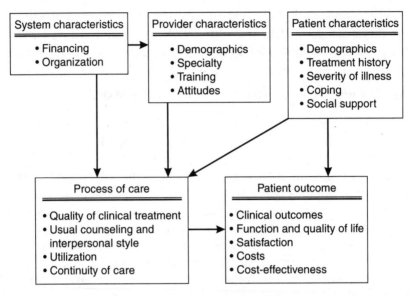

Figure 4.1   Depression Care Evaluation Framework

ganization and financing that apply across systems or contrast overall differences through a few discrete characteristics. The former approach can provide more information on which components are important, but it is expensive and often limited to a case-study approach that has little generalizability. The latter strategy is less expensive and provides an overall summary, but it largely leaves each system as a "black box." We generally contrast types of financing systems (PP versus FFS) and only occasionally open the black box by assessing the organization of the delivery system (HMOs, multispecialty groups, solo practices), the perceived generosity of coverage for mental health services, and the practice characteristics (group size, staffing, including mix of physicians and nonphysicians and of primary care and specialty physicians).

Patient Characteristics: Casemix and Outcomes

Patient characteristics, often referred to as "casemix" in health services research, provide statistical controls to reduce selection biases in observational studies. The MOS developed a comprehensive set of measures of patient sociodemographic and health characteristics that might predict quality or outcomes of care. Not all studies can afford a similarly detailed measurement framework. Researchers thus need to pay particular attention to factors that are most likely to bias results for their questions in the design phase and select measures and analytic strategies accordingly.

The common, although arbitrary, distinction between health outcomes and casemix addresses this design issue. If all aspects of health status related to a condition such as depression could be identified and measured, this distinction would become irrelevant, as one could measure all aspects of health status over time and estimate (through panel data analysis) how treatment affects changes in health status over time. Such a comprehensive measurement is infeasible; every study must select some aspects of health status that are of primary interest and that become "outcomes." Baseline assessments of outcomes are only a part of casemix, however, as other dimensions of health status predict outcomes of interest or processes of care. The MOS considered some components of health status, such as number of symptoms or functioning, to be outcomes and measured them at baseline and follow-up interviews, whereas it considered others, such as comorbidities, solely components of casemix. In the next chapter we will discuss health outcomes measurement in detail.

In clinical trials of depression, the strongest predictors of depression status over time are baseline number and intensity of symptoms of depression, the presence of melancholia, and previous spells of depression. We included a history of two or more prior spells of depression as a marker of recurrent depression, which predicts relapse probability and indicates continued use of antidepressant medication to prevent recurrence. We did not determine the recency of prior spells and so could not apply the Depression Guidelines Panel's (1993b) recency criteria as an indicator of the necessity of maintenance therapy.

Psychiatric comorbidities can complicate the assessment or treatment of depression, making them an important component of casemix. The MOS included two that were common and easy to measure: concurrent anxiety disorder (panic disorder, generalized anxiety disorder, simple phobia, and psychotic symptoms) and alcohol and drug abuse. Concurrent anxiety disorders must be assessed to determine which type of disorder (anxiety or depression) is primary (Depression Guidelines Panel, 1993a). Psychotic symptoms could indicate psychotic depression (which may require hospitalization or antipsychotic medications) or, in the recent DSM classification, a disorder that precludes a diagnosis of major depressive disorder. Substance abuse disorder is likely to require treatment before depression can be treated successfully (Regier et al., 1990; Schuckit, 1986). There are many other comorbidities, including DSM-III Axis I disorders and Axis II (personality) disorders, that we could not include because we did not have the resources for clinical assessments, and brief screening measures were unavailable. For example, there were no well-validated screening measures for personality disorders when the study was designed.

Medical comorbidities can also complicate the assessment or treatment of depression (Rodin, Craven, and Littlefield, 1991). The MOS assessed the most common chronic conditions for which patients seek health care, including hypertension, diabetes type I and II, myocardial infarction, congestive heart failure, arthritis, and chronic lung conditions. Because patients also seek care for acute symptoms that are not disease specific (sleep problems, pain, gastrointestinal or respiratory symptoms), it is useful to include brief measures of such symptoms. To account for the many other health problems that exist, one approach uses a multidimensional assessment of health-related quality of life, such as the SF-36 (Ware and Sherbourne, 1992), which was developed for the MOS, as a general control for other psychiatric and medical comorbid conditions and symptoms.

Psychosocial risk and protective factors address a different dimension of casemix. These factors include patient attitudes regarding the importance of depression and acceptability of depression treatment; occurrence of stressful life events; amount and quality of social support; and psychological coping style, especially active versus passive modes of coping with stress. Attitudes toward depression care may affect utilization patterns or adherence to treatment recommendations (Leaf, Bruce, and Tischler, 1986); stressful life events may serve as a risk factor for subsequent illness; and strong social support may buffer the negative impact of stressful life events and protect against future depression (Billings, Cronkite, and Moos, 1983; George et al., 1989; Moos, 1990; Sherbourne and Hays, 1990).

Although sociodemographic factors are generally considered part of casemix, we distinguish between patient factors that are potentially endogenous to the condition of depression (such as income) and factors that are exogenous (such as ethnicity). Endogenous factors are directly affected by the condition or causally linked to it (depression can lead to unemployment and reduced income) and may therefore become an outcome; exogenous factors are causally independent. Whether or not a factor is endogenous often depends on the research question posed. For adolescents or young adults, educational achievement could be affected by depression; and marital status and even family size could be endogenous in a long-run study if symptoms of depression precipitate a separation or divorce. In a short-run analysis, however, such as a study of acute-phase treatment of major depressive disorder, the same demographic factors are unlikely to be affected by changes in health status.

Provider Characteristics

Clinicians determine processes of care with patients, and differences in clinician characteristics (such as training) could lead to observed differences in performance of different health care delivery systems. For example, older and younger clinicians may have different levels of skill in assessing depression (Robbins et al., 1994), and generalist and specialty internists differ in intensity of preventive counseling activities (Wells, Lewis, Leake, Schleiter, and Brook, 1986). Studying clinician characteristics allows one to explore the reasons for differences between health care systems and isolates clinician factors from financial incentives and other system characteristics. This may be particularly important for designing clinical interventions that focus on improving quality of care. The main clinician characteristics studied in the MOS were specialty (primary care, medical subspecialty, psychiatry, psychology, master's-level therapist), age, ethnicity, gender, exposure to continuing education experiences (including seminars on depression), and fellowship training (including psychoanalytic training).

The Design of the MOS

The MOS examined care for patients with hypertension, heart disease (coronary heart disease, congestive heart failure), diabetes (early-

and late-onset), and depression. The overall design has previously been described by Rogers et al. (1992) and Tarlov et al. (1989); details on data collection can be found in Berry (1992); and details on the longitudinal design for the depression component are included in Rogers et al. (1993) and Wells et al. (1992).

Site and Provider Selection

The MOS study sites were selected for geographic diversity. To qualify as a study site, a city had to have an HMO with a minimum of 100,000 enrollees and large multispecialty group practices (MSGs) with at least 10 physicians that had been in operation for at least three years. The three final sites, chosen from twelve candidate sites, were Boston, Chicago, and Los Angeles.

Within each site, the MOS selected a representative sample of clinicians from HMOs, MSGs, and small group and solo practices (SOLO), including general internists, family practitioners, cardiologists, endocrinologists, psychiatrists, psychologists, and (in group practices only) master's-level mental health specialists who practiced independently. Eligible clinicians had practiced in their settings for at least three years, were between the ages of thirty-one and fifty-five (to standardize age range across specialty), were not primarily involved in governmental practice (for example, Veterans Administration or military), and did not have predominantly non-English-speaking patients.

The participating HMOs and MSGs had 266 eligible clinicians, of whom 225 (85 percent) agreed to participate. In the SOLO practices, a multistage selection process was used, including stratified random sampling from lists provided by national professional associations, followed by further screening for eligibility and willingness to participate. At the final stage, 491 eligible clinicians agreed to consider enrolling in the study, and 298 (61 percent) actually enrolled. Although SOLO clinician participation rates were low, there was no significant bias related to clinician demographic, training, or practice characteristics. The total MOS sample included 523 participating clinicians, about 21 percent of whom were women; the majority (85 percent) of participants were white, with 4 percent African American, 3 percent Latino, and 7 percent Asian American.

Sampling Patients

Within the practices of participating clinicians, patients were asked to complete a self-administered questionnaire. Seventy-five percent of the eligible patients in HMO and MSG practices and 65 percent in SOLO practices completed the screening form between March and October 1986, for a total of 22,399 adult outpatients. In addition, the clinicians completed an encounter form for each screening visit.

All HMO, SOLO, and MSG practices included patients receiving PP care; PP patients in SOLO and MSG practices were considered members of independent practice association (IPA) plans. In addition, the SOLO and MSG practices also had patients receiving FFS care. The percentage of patients with PP coverage was 100 percent in HMOs, about 50 percent in MSGs, and about 15 percent in the SOLO sector.

Identifying Depressed Patients

The study did not require that depressed patients be in treatment specifically for depression, and identification for depression used a two-stage screener, independent of whether or not patients' providers were aware of their depression and whether or not patients were seeking care for depression. The first-stage depression screener was an eight-item depression-symptom scale (six items from the Center for Epidemiologic Studies' Depression Scale, or CES-D, two from the Diagnostic Interview Schedule, or DIS) that elicits information on intensity of depression symptoms (for example, feeling sad or crying spells) over the past week and on periods of depressed mood over the past year (see Appendix C). Burnam et al. (1988) developed a scoring algorithm for the eight items and identified a cutoff score that has excellent sensitivity (86–92 percent across different primary care and mental health specialty outpatient samples) and acceptable positive predictive value (20–37 percent in primary care outpatient samples, 48–50 percent in mental health specialty outpatient samples) for identifying persons who have current (one-year) DSM-III depressive disorder, that is, major depression and / or dysthymia. The second-stage screening instrument was the depression section of the National Institute of Mental Health Diagnostic Interview Schedule (DIS) (Robins et al., 1981), a highly structured diagnostic assessment tool administered by a lay person that includes supplemental questions assessing the full DSM-III criteria of major depression, dysthymia, and melancholia. The second-stage telephone screen took place between May and December 1986.

Of those screened, 2,194 patients exceeded the first-stage screener cut-point, were study-eligible, and completed the second-stage screening with the DIS. Of those, 1,772 were enrolled in the longitudinal phase of the study. Among patients eligible for the second-stage depression screening, those completing the interview were significantly more educated (by one-half a year on average), more likely to be married (47 percent versus 39 percent), and less likely to be male (28 percent versus 31 percent). Also, response rates were higher in the group practices than the SOLO sector. Diabetics had higher response rates, and individuals with higher depression-symptom screener scores (higher probabilities of having current depressive disorder) were somewhat less likely to respond.

Patients exceeding the depression-symptoms screener cut-point for high probability of having depressive disorder were defined as having *depressive symptoms.* This cut-point is equivalent to having a 35 percent probability of current depressive disorder in general medical practices and a 50 percent probability in mental health specialty practices. Those with current major depression or dysthymia, according to the criteria of the DSM-III, were defined as having *current depressive disorder* (those with both types of disorder are referred to as having "double depression," after Keller, Lavori, Endicott, Coryell, and Klerman, 1983). Given that lifetime criteria for major depression were met, we relaxed the definition of current major depression to include persons with three or more (rather than four or more) DSM-III Criteria B symptom groups, based on recommendations in Helzer et al. (1985), to increase the sensitivity of the DIS in identifying major depression. Only 43 patients entered the study as a result of this relaxation of the criteria. Of the 2,194 who were eligible for and completed the telephone DIS, 35 percent ($N = 772$) met study criteria for current depressive disorder. Persons with depressive symptoms but no current disorder are considered to have *subthreshold depression,* but among them we distinguish between persons with lifetime (that is, past) depressive disorder and those with no history of depressive disorder.

Patients meeting study criteria for depression were asked to participate in a more detailed health assessment, in which their functioning and well-being, prior use of services, profile of lifetime and recent psychiatric disorders, severity of depression, and medical comorbidities were assessed through a series of structured interviews or self-report questionnaires. Because different components of the assessment were given at different times and by different methods of administration (telephone-administered, self-administered, clinician-elicited history), the sample sizes vary for different components of the assessment.

A probability sample was then selected for the longitudinal study. By design, the elderly (those over sixty-five) were oversampled. All eligible patients with heart disease and current depressive disorder were selected for the panel, along with a 50 percent random sample of those with depressive symptoms but no current disorder. Because the health outcome measures at baseline were included in the Patient Assessment Questionnaire (PAQ), PAQ response was a high priority in panel selection. Of the 1,772 enrolled depressed patients, 974 were selected for the longitudinal panel. We estimate a refusal or nonresponse rate of 28 percent (Wells et al., 1992).

Collecting Outcomes and Use Data

All patients in the longitudinal portion of the MOS (not just the depression panel) were asked to complete self-administered questionnaires at six-month intervals for two follow-up years, and then again at four years of follow-up. Among depressed patients, 69–70 percent responded to the follow-up self-report PAQs, and patients who were initially more depressed were less likely to respond.

In addition, patients with lifetime (or at a level just missing lifetime criteria) or current depressive disorder were also contacted for a structured, computer-assisted telephone interview (the Course of Depression (COD) interview, Wells et al., 1992) to obtain information on course of depression, use of psychotropic medications, and functioning outcomes. The first wave of the COD interviews took place in October and November 1987, the second wave in October and November 1988. For the 771 eligible patients (not everybody in the longitudinal panel was eligible), 74–75 percent responded to each wave, with 617 (83 percent) responding to at least one COD. Regarding response bias, the respondents to the first follow-up COD were more likely to have diabetes, to be white, married, female, and to have lower first-stage depression-screener scores. On the second follow-up COD, respondents were more likely to be married, but other factors were unrelated to response.

Throughout the study, we analyzed nonresponse and attrition at each step of baseline assessment and longitudinal follow-up. To make results refer to a common reference population, most (but not all) analyses weight the data to the full screener sample eligible for the depression component of the study.

Patient Characteristics

The average age in the full longitudinal sample was forty-four years; 70 percent of the patients were female and 47 percent were married. On average, the sample had one year of college, but patients of psychiatrists had on average one to two years more of college. Sixty-one percent were employed, but this percentage was as high as 81 percent in FFS psychology and as low as 46 percent in FFS psychiatry. Ethnic minorities composed 22 percent of the sample, but this percentage was lower in mental health specialty practices.

Provider Characteristics

The average age in the clinician sample ($N = 523$) was forty years; only about one in five clinicians was female. There were significantly more nonwhite clinicians in general medical practices (15 percent) than in mental health specialty practices (10 percent in psychiatry, 3 percent in psychology). Patient volume was more than twice as high in general medicine, where only 52 percent were solo practitioners, than in mental health specialty, where 70 percent were solo practitioners.

Chapter Five

Measuring Quality of Care and Outcomes

Monitoring costs, quality of care, and health outcomes is necessary to determine the performance of a health care delivery setting. Such performance evaluations are already required, although to a limited extent, by some employer organizations buying health insurance. They will increase in scope and importance as buyers realize that price is not the only determinant of value and that health benefits can be compared.

Despite much current interest in evaluating the performance of health plans and practices, however, many practitioners and researchers do not know how best to measure performance. In this chapter we discuss the main measures of processes of care and health outcomes for depression used in the MOS and provide suggestions about how to select among measures. The details necessary to score and use those measures are given in Appendixes A and B. Appendix C provides additional descriptive statistics from the MOS, which can be used as a benchmark for comparisons.

Process of Care

The process components in the MOS bridge clinical and health services research but emphasize treatments of established efficacy: quality of clinical treatments for depression; clinician usual counseling and interpersonal style of care; and use of mental health services and continuity of care.

59

Quality of Clinical Treatments for Depression

The evaluation of quality of clinical care is based on a model of sequential treatment steps (Figure 5.1) similar to the models in Wells (1985) and the Depression Guidelines Panel (1993a, b). Initial clinician detection or awareness of patient depression triggers a fuller clinical assessment. Clinicians and patients then select a treatment method. We focus on antidepressant medications, counseling (as a proxy for psychotherapy), and referral to another provider as the predominant treatments for outpatients. The clinician monitors adherence to treatment recommendations and response to treatment through follow-up visits (continuity of care), which can include continuation and maintenance therapy. Merely listing these steps does not yield a measurement approach. The necessary tasks include developing operational definitions of each step, selecting the level of clinical precision and comprehensiveness, and developing the corre-

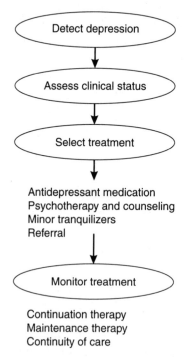

Figure 5.1   Steps in Care for Depression

sponding measures. A study must often compromise between breadth (range of processes) and depth (clinical precision for each process), depending on study questions and resources. For the MOS, the priority was to measure components associated with health outcomes, especially for the acute phase of treatment. Table 5.1 summarizes our clinical treatment measures.

Detection

A post-visit form filled out by the clinicians asked whether the patient had a clinically meaningful depression lasting at least two weeks during the past year and whether another clinician was treating the patient for depression. The MOS compared the clinician report with the study's independent assessment. Because some clinicians may not formally detect depression, we permitted an "implicit" recognition of depression by asking the clinicians if:

1. depression, anxiety, or some other emotional or family problem was the main cause of the visit;
2. counseling for three minutes or more occurred for each of these problems; and
3. the patient was referred to a mental health specialist.

We analyzed four increasingly broad definitions of detection. The most restrictive definition is formal recognition of depression; a more general definition ("depression visit") requires either formal recognition, listing depression as a main reason for the visit, or counseling for depression. An even broader definition ("mental health visit") includes the above—listing either anxiety as a main reason for the visit or providing counseling for depression—or referring the patient to a mental health specialist. The broadest definition ("psychosocial visit") includes the above or listing either any emotional or family problem as the reason for the visit or providing counseling for the problem. Although as the definition broadens a higher percentage of patients are identified as detected, specialty and payment conclusions are not sensitive to this method's effect. Thus policy studies probably need only the narrow definition, but studies more focused on absolute levels of care, such as quality improvement studies, may need broader definitions.

Table 5.1   Clinical Treatment

Measure	Definition
Detection of depression	
Detection of depression	Provider aware during the visit that the patient had "two weeks or more of a clinically meaningful depression during the previous twelve months"
Depression visit	Provider listed the main reason for the office visit as depression or counseled the patient about depression during the visit
Mental health visit	Provider listed the main reason for the office visit as depression or another psychiatric problem, counseled the patient about depression or anxiety, or referred the patient to a mental health specialist during the visit
Psychosocial visit	Provider listed the main reason for the office visit as any psychiatric mental or psychosocial problem, counseled the patient about any psychiatric, personal, family, or emotional problem, or referred the patient to a mental health specialist during the visit
Counseling for depression	
Counseled for depression	Provider counseled the patient for three minutes or more for depression during the visit
Quality and use of psychotropic medications	
Used antidepressants	Patient reported using an antidepressant medication daily, for at least a month, during the prior six months, regardless of dosage, or used ever in the prior month
Effective use of antidepressants	Use of an effective dosage (i.e., equivalent to 75 mg. or more daily of imipramine for the nonelderly, and 50 mg. or more daily for the elderly) among all depressed patients
Used minor tranquilizers	Patient reported using a tranquilizer medication daily, for at least a month, during the prior six months, regardless of dosage, or used ever in the prior month

Table 5.1   (continued)

Measure	Definition
Unmet need	
Unmet need for care of depression	Patient reported needing care for depression but did not receive care (among those reporting problems in the past six months)
Unmet need for care of psychosocial problems	Patient reported needing care for depression, family or marital problems, alcohol or drug problems, sexual problems or concerns, or other personal, emotional, behavioral, or mental problems
Appropriate care	
Appropriate care for depression	Depression was detected and the patient was either counseled or referred to a mental health specialist during the visit or some other clinician was noted as providing the majority of care for depression
Referral	
Referral to mental health specialty care	Provider referred the patient to a mental health specialist during the visit

Quality of Psychotropic Medication Use

There are difficult issues in measuring medication use, as patient self-report is often considered unreliable and pharmacy data may not reflect actual use. Strategies to increase reliability and validity include direct observation of medication containers, interviews by clinicians, direct measurement of medication levels, and so on. In the MOS, study clinicians interviewed patients about their medications over the telephone or in person and requested information (number of days of use in the last month and daily dosage) about each medication used in the prior month or used daily for emotional or personal problems for at least a month during the prior six months.[1] At baseline, study clinicians compared medication containers and pictures of medications from the Physician's Desk Reference to confirm reports.

For each antidepressant medication, we determined whether or not the daily dosage was below recommended minimum therapeutic levels (Katon et al., 1992; Wells et al., 1994). We obtained information on minor tranquilizer dosages, but we used only an indicator variable of any use in the assessment period.

Unmet Need

Unmet need is commonly considered a component of access (that is, for general populations) but can also apply to users who have not been helped for a particular problem. The measures of unmet need (a narrow definition of unmet need for depression care and a broader definition of unmet need for help with any emotional or personal problem) are based on patient report at baseline. In the MOS, unmet need meant that a patient reported needing help for depression or any emotional or personal problem but did not receive it.

Appropriate Care

Care at the baseline visit was defined as appropriate if the depression was detected and there was some evidence of treatment (counseling, listing depression as a main reason for the visit, or noting that another clinician provided care for depression). Care was defined as equivocal if there was evidence of detection but no treatment, or vice versa. Inappropriate care was defined as having a depression that was neither detected nor treated. The advantage of this concept over a measure of detection or treatment alone is that it gives extra credit to providers with more complete treatment strategies.

Referral

Clinicians reported whether or not the patient was referred to a mental health specialist during a visit in which the patient was acutely depressed.

Counseling

Counseling is the most difficult process to measure because general medical providers are likely to discount their own advice and education and not report it as "therapy." Yet their counseling may differ qualitatively from that provided by mental health specialists. Although we were not optimistic that we could capture the effects of counseling in the MOS, we developed a simple measure of exposure to minimal counseling: clinicians were asked whether they provided three minutes or more of face-to-face counseling for depression, anxiety, or personal, emotional, and family problems during an index visit. Independently, patients were asked to describe the kind of counseling they received (group, individual, family / marital, or other therapy) from specialists in the prior six months.

Usual Clinician Counseling and Interpersonal Style

These counseling indicator variables are very limited direct measures of counseling that obscure differences among specialists and render counseling a "black box." We complemented them with clinician-level measures of counseling and interpersonal style (defined in Table 5.2), an extension of the framework of Wells et al. (1984a, b) for assessing health promotion activities and the work of Kaplan, Greenfield, and Ware (1989) on aspects of physician-patient interactions that predict outcomes in chronic disease. The *counseling style* domains include the likelihood of the clinician's initiating and providing counseling, the duration (or intensity) of counseling, the types of techniques usually applied, and the perceived skill in counseling (based on the Health Belief Model, Rosenstock, 1974).

Clinicians rated at baseline their level of counseling initiative (how routinely they initiate counseling) and perceived skill when counseling patients about four issues: (1) marital or family problems; (2) depression; (3) sexual functioning; and (4) coping with physical illness or symptoms. To measure preferences for counseling, clinicians rated the likelihood of their providing counseling for patients with depression and no comorbid chronic medical illness, and depression co-occurring with myocardial infarction, hypertension, or diabetes.[2] Intensity of counseling was measured by asking clinicians how much time they usually spent when counseling, and responses were dichotomized to

Table 5.2   Clinician Usual Counseling Style and Interpersonal Style

Measure	Definition/item content
Counseling style	
Initiative	Whether and extent to which clinician usually raises issue for discussion with patients
	Marital or family problems
	Depression
	Sexual functioning
	Coping with physical illness or symptoms
Perceived skill	Perceptions of skill in counseling patients
	Marital or family problems
	Depression
	Sexual functioning
	Coping with physical illness or symptoms
Preference for depression counseling	Likelihood of providing ongoing (three or more visits) face-to-face counseling to treat moderate to severe depression for different patient groups
	Depression, no major medical illness
	Depression and recent myocardial infarction
	Depression and hypertension
	Depression and diabetes
Intensity (duration)	Amount of visit time taken to deal with emotional issues or patients' personal problems
Technique	Usual technique used in face-to-face counseling of patients for personal, emotional, or family problems
	Education or advice
	Interpretations or confrontations
	Counseling family members
	Behavioral treatments (e.g., relaxation or stress management)
	Psychodynamic therapy
	Did not personally counsel
Interpersonal style	
Egalitarian participation	Extent to which clinician conveys a sense of dominance, directiveness, judgmentalness, and impression of authority to patients
	Good doctors use their authority to shape patient behavior
	Treatment recommendations presented with authority are more likely to be accepted by patients

Table 5.2   (continued)

Measure	Definition/item content
	Among competent professionals, those who maintain a strong air of authority usually obtain the best results in treating patients
	Sometimes it is best to pressure patients to get them to do what is best for them
Share treatment decision-making	Tendency for clinician to share control with the patient regarding treatment decisions
	I prefer that patients leave decisions about their treatment up to me
	If I make patients feel that they are making treatment choices themselves, their disease management is better
	It is best to let patients participate in decisions whenever choices between treatment options are available
	Most patients are unable to make intelligent choices about their care

distinguish clinicians who did and did not spend more than ten minutes counseling. Counseling techniques were assessed by asking clinicians which procedures they used when counseling (that is, education or advice; interpretations or confrontations; counseling family members; behavioral treatments; and psychodynamic therapy).

Interpersonal style domains likely to be related to counseling are egalitarian participation style and style of sharing treatment decisions. Egalitarian participation style or level of authority in the patient-clinician relationship was assessed with four items, as was the tendency for clinicians to share control over treatment decisions with patients. Appendix B presents scoring rules for each style measure. All are coded on a 0–100 scale, with higher scores consistent with the direction of the scale name.

Evaluation of Counseling Style Measures

Table 5.3 provides descriptive statistics for counseling style measures by clinician specialty.

Table 5.3 Characteristics of Clinician Usual Counseling and Interpersonal Style of Care Measures

Measure	No. of items	Mean	SD	Reliability	Item-total correlations	Floor (%)	Ceiling (%)	Complete data (%)
Mental health specialists								
Counseling style								
Initiative	4	47.7	20.0	.89	.72–85	0	0	90
Perceived skill	4	65.5	8.6	.45	.25–32	0	0	93
Preference for depression counseling	4	95.7	11.5	.90	.72–91	1	71	92
Intensity (duration)	1	100.0[a]	0.0	N.A.	N.A.	N.A.	N.A.	N.A.
Interpersonal style								
Egalitarian participation	4	49.7	16.3	.63	.33–49	0	1	93
Share treatment decision-making	4	81.9	13.3	.60	.31–50	0	13	93
General medical clinicians								
Counseling style								
Initiative	4	43.7	12.1	.62	.14–45	<1	0	88
Perceived skill	4	40.1	14.3	.78	.48–68	<1	0	88
Preference for depression counseling	4	52.9	35.0	.96	.80–95	14	10	76
Intensity (duration)	1	44.8	49.8	N.A.	N.A.	N.A.	N.A.	N.A.
Interpersonal style								
Egalitarian participation	4	47.6	14.9	.61	.33–44	0	0	88
Share treatment decision-making	4	74.7	14.0	.62	.34–48	0	5	88

Note: All measures were scaled from 0 to 100 in the direction indicated by their name. N.A. = Not Applicable.
a. All mental health specialists counseled for ten minutes or more.

A standard criterion for evaluating the psychometric properties of a multi-item scale is *reliability,* which refers to the proportion of information that a score contains, as opposed to random error. Our reliability measure is *internal consistency,* or the extent to which multiple items in a scale measure the same underlying concept (Cronbach, 1951). All scales of clinician usual style of care are sufficiently reliable to compare groups of physicians among general medical providers or mental health specialists, but they should not be used to compare individual clinicians, with the possible exception of preference for counseling depression. Among mental health specialists, the scale for perceived skill has very low reliability, so we would recommend further development and testing of this scale before its use in other applications.[3] The scale that measures the clinician's preference for providing face-to-face counseling for depression showed a high degree of clustering at the high end of the scale distribution among mental health specialists, as one might expect, given that this is a common form of treatment provided by these clinicians. Thus this measure may be most useful when describing typical general medical practices rather than mental health specialty providers.

Aside from reliability, it is also important to know how well the clinician style measures reflect actual clinician behavior. We examined their *predictive validity*[4] by comparing usual style scales with actual treatment, including quality of clinical treatments, face-to-face visit time, and patient satisfaction with the visit.[5]

Contrasting clinicians scoring at the twenty-fifth and the seventy-fifth percentile values of each style scale, we found that higher clinician counseling preference was significantly associated with better quality of care: higher rates of detection, counseling, and mental health specialty referral (among general medical providers), although the differences in rates were not very large. Higher perceived counseling skill was associated with higher rates of detection and higher patient satisfaction. More egalitarian participation style was associated with higher detection, counseling, and more overall appropriate care for depression. Some comparisons for other scales were significant, but could be due to chance.[6] Overall, it appears that preference for counseling is a reliable scale that predicts treatment well; the other scales may not be as useful and should not be used as substitutes for direct patient-level measures of quality of clinical treatment until further scale development has been performed.

Utilization and Continuity of Care

Use of services is a standard health services research perspective on process of care and includes access to care over time and level of care. The MOS relied exclusively on patient self-report, not medical record abstraction or computerized data, to estimate hospitalization and visit rates over time, and utilization items were repeated on every follow-up questionnaire.

The MOS did not contribute much new information regarding measurement of service use and costs. Therefore, we do not include additional statistics and measures in the appendix for utilization. There are three issues that deserve attention, however: (1) distinguishing causes of visits from the patient's perspective; (2) studying provider and health care plan continuity; and (3) using visit data for case-mix adjustment.

We distinguish between visits for mental health reasons and visits for medical reasons from the patient's perspective. Every visit that a patient reported for mental health reasons was counted as a mental health visit, regardless of the type of provider. It is important to measure mental health utilization this way because many depressed patients receive all their care in the general medical sector. Studies that cannot distinguish between mental health and medical reasons for a visit, and instead classify visits according to provider type, are likely to find a spurious "cost-offset" effect because patients of mental health specialists have fewer visits to general medical providers than patients receiving their mental health care in the general medical sector.

We studied continuity of care by tracking whether or not the patient was still seeing the initial MOS clinician over time. Discontinuities in care relationships for sick patients could be associated with worse outcomes, and continuity may therefore be a quality-of-care measure. Research on depression has not focused on continuity in this more general sense, but continuity is an important component of case management strategies for seriously mentally ill populations in the public sector (Bachrach, 1993). Although we did not develop this continuity measure to use as a component of quality of care, we now believe that this is an important quality-of-care component to assess. In addition, we measured the continuity of insurance status to track switches between payment systems.

In the absence of clinical data, many studies have used prior use of services as a component of casemix to measure the need for services. This is not an adequate strategy for studying the effect of payment system or provider specialty on utilization, because prior use is endogenous to payment system and provider specialty. We generally avoided utilization as a proxy for health and instead controlled directly for baseline health status.

Outcomes of Care

The MOS analyses of depression outcomes focused almost exclusively on the health measures discussed in this section, but economic consequences are also important outcomes of health care. Economic consequences are not only treatment costs (largely a health plan perspective) but indirect economic effects, such as income and wealth changes for patients and family members that result from the impact of depression and its treatment. These income and wealth changes may be related to missed work for health care visits or poor work performance. Such indirect effects are likely to be far more important for evaluating health care for depression from a social perspective than direct treatment costs (Greenberg et al., 1993).

The MOS studied health outcomes primarily from the patient's point of view through patient self-report, an approach recommended by many medical and research leaders (Ellwood, 1988; Geigle and Jones, 1990; Tarlov et al., 1989; Ware, 1992, 1993a). We distinguished two types of health outcomes: (1) clinical status; and (2) health-related quality of life (HRQOL), or daily functioning and well-being. Satisfaction with care is sometimes considered an outcome—in some studies, it is even the only outcome evaluated—but we consider it a proxy measure for quality of care. We found that satisfaction has some predictive ability for counseling and medication use, but—in contrast with counseling and antidepressant medication—satisfaction has no significant and qualitatively robust relationship with improved functioning over time among any patient group. Thus we consider satisfaction less useful for studying quality of care than direct process or health measures and do not discuss it further. Satisfaction may be a useful measure for limited studies that cannot afford to measure processes of care or health outcomes, however. Satisfaction may also be an important predictor of a health plan's economic success, as disenrollment will decrease as satisfaction increases, regardless of the actual clinical quality of care. We also found that satisfaction predicts the probability that patients will switch providers.

Clinical Status

The clinical status outcomes, including remission, new episode, and symptoms, are defined in Table 5.4 (Keller et al., 1982; Keller, Lavori, Lewis, and Klerman, 1983; Kupfer, 1991). Depressive symptoms (number, intensity) are the most common outcomes in clinical trials. Remission and new episode are outcomes that apply to patient subgroups. Descriptive statistics by type of depression and specialty of treating provider are included in Appendix C.

Clinical outcomes were assessed with the COD interview, a computer-assisted telephone interview modeled on the format of the DIS (Wells et al., 1992).[7] We used a count of symptoms (up to thirty) of major depression, dysthymia, and melancholia over the prior year, which affords a uniform outcome measure across diagnostic groups (see Table 5.5). This measure includes most of the symptoms in more traditional clinical trial measures (The Hamilton Depression Rating Scale, the Beck Depression Inventory) but has the advantage of being scored directly from the diagnostic measure.[8] We identified any remission of major depressive episodes during a follow-up year, and incidence or new episode of major depressive disorder among patients with subthreshold depression or dysthymia only at baseline.[9]

Table 5.4 Definition of Clinical Measures

Measure	Definition
Remission	Eight weeks or more with two or fewer symptoms of depression among those with major depression at baseline
New episode	A new episode of major depression among those without current major depression at baseline
Symptoms	Number of symptoms (out of thirty) of major depression or dysthymia during a given period

Table 5.5   Depressive Symptoms

Two weeks or more of feeling sad, depressed, uninterested in things
Felt depressed or sad most days
Work (at home or on the job) suffered
Lost ability to enjoy being paid a compliment
Lost ability to feel better even after hearing good news
Became cross or irritable when depressed
Troubled by a period of crying spells
Lost appetite for two weeks or longer
Lost weight without trying—two lbs./wk. for several weeks
Eating increased—gained two lbs./wk. for several weeks
Had trouble falling asleep, staying asleep, or woke too early
Slept too much
Woke up two hours early
Felt tired out all the time
Felt very bad when you first got up
Talked or moved more slowly than normal
Had to be moving all the time
Felt fidgety or restless most of the time
Interest in sex was a lot less than usual
Lost all interest in things like work, hobbies, things you usually like to do
   for fun
Wanted to stay away from people
Felt worthless, sinful, or guilty
Had little self-confidence
Felt life was hopeless or pointless
Had a lot more trouble concentrating than is normal
Thoughts came much more slowly than usual
Thought a lot about death
Felt like you wanted to die
Thought of committing suicide
Attempted suicide

Health-Related Quality of Life (HRQOL)

The main outcome for the MOS was morbidity, or HRQOL. The MOS measurement of HRQOL is documented in the book *Measuring Functioning and Well-Being: The Medical Outcomes Study Approach* (Stewart and Ware, 1992). The central definition of health followed the World Health Organization (WHO, 1948), which emphasizes physical, mental, and social well-being, not just the absence of diseases. The MOS adaptation of the WHO framework emphasized physical and mental health more than social well-being (Figure 5.2) because of controversy over the latter construct's status as a component of health (Donald and Ware, 1982; Ware, 1986). Social functioning and well-being are central outcomes for depression (Weissman and Klerman, 1992), however.

Empirically, physical and mental domains of health overlap (Hays and Stewart, 1990), and the clinical and theoretical distinction between physical and mental health problems is somewhat artificial. For example, physical symptoms and underlying biological causes apply to depression as well as chronic medical conditions. Despite this artificiality, we refer to the larger constructs of health in our HRQOL model as "physical" and "mental" health domains to be consistent with the literature.

The central concepts of HRQOL, *functioning* and *well-being,* are relevant to both mental and physical constructs. Functioning refers to people's ability to perform their daily tasks and activities (for example, climbing stairs, walking a mile, taking frequent rests at work) (Stewart and Kamberg, 1992), whereas well-being refers to more subjective internal states, such as experiencing bodily pain or anxiety (Sherbourne, 1992a). The HRQOL domains, defined in Table 5.6,

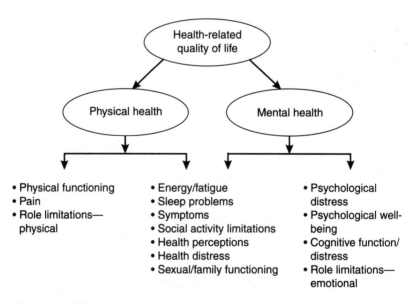

Figure 5.2   Health-Related Quality of Life

Table 5.6 Definitions of Health-Related Quality-of-Life (HRQOL) Domains

Domain	Definition
Functioning	
Physical	Limitations due to health in activities such as sports, climbing stairs, walking, dressing, and bathing
Serious limitations	Current limitations in vigorous and moderate activities and inability to work around the house or at a paying job
Role–physical	Extent to which physical health problems interfere with doing work or other regular daily activities in last four weeks
Role–emotional	Extent to which emotional problems interfere with doing work or other regular daily activities in last four weeks
Social	Extent to which health interferes with social activities such as visiting friends or relatives in the past month
Cognitive	Amount of time in past month spent confused, reacting slowly to things, having difficulty reasoning
Bed days	Number of days in bed due to health in the last thirty days
Sexual	Extent of sexual problems during the past four weeks
Marital	Relationship with spouse or partner over the past four weeks (closeness, supportiveness, sharing)
Well-being	
General health	Perceptions of overall current health, health outlook, and resistance to illness in general
Bodily pain	Extent of bodily pain in the past four weeks
Mental health	General mood or affect, including depression, anxiety, and positive well-being in the last month
Energy/fatigue	Amount of time in last four weeks spent feeling energetic versus tired and worn out
Sleep problems	Sleep disturbance, adequacy, somnolence, and shortness of breath on awakening during the past four weeks
Symptoms	Frequency of seven common physical and psychophysiologic symptoms, such as stiffness, coughing, nausea, acid indigestion, heavy feelings in arms or legs, headaches, and backaches in past four weeks

were assessed using different specific self-report measures, such as long-form instruments that afford greater precision or one of several short-form measures that provide feasible alternatives in busy clinical practice settings (Hays, Sherbourne, and Mazel, 1993; Hays and Stewart, 1990; Sherbourne, 1992a, b, c; Sherbourne, Allen, Kamberg, and Wells, 1992; Sherbourne and Kamberg, 1992; Sherbourne, Stewart, and Wells, 1992; Stewart, Hays, and Ware, 1992; Stewart and Kamberg, 1992; Stewart and Ware, 1992; Stewart, Ware, Sherbourne, and Wells, 1992; Ware and Sherbourne, 1992; and Ware, Sherbourne, and Davies, 1992).

Evaluation of HRQOL Measures for Depression

We selected fourteen measures from the more than seventy developed for the MOS as a recommended strategy for future evaluations of depressed patients. These selected measures represent primary symptoms of depression or target goals of treatment, correlated physical symptoms, or policy-relevant physical and role problems that afford comparisons with chronic medical conditions. They include the eight SF-36 measures (Ware and Sherbourne, 1992), but we applied the RAND 36-Item Health Survey scoring rules for two subscales (Hays, Sherbourne, and Mazel, 1993); a measure of serious role-physical limitations that proved to be particularly useful in the depression analyses for this book (Rogers et al., 1993); and five full-length MOS measures not otherwise included in short-form measures.

The reliability and validity of many MOS short-form measures have received support in several studies in the United States and Europe (Brazier et al., 1992; Jenkinson et al., 1993; McHorney et al., 1992, 1994; Ware, Sherbourne, and Davies, 1992), and general population norms are available for comparative purposes (McHorney et al., 1994; Ware, 1993b; Ware, Sherbourne, and Davies, 1992). Less is known, however, about how well these measures perform for depressed patients. Descriptive statistics on these fourteen measures, based on data from the 974 depressed patients in the MOS longitudinal patient sample, are provided in Table 5.7.[10] Because scales differ in the number and levels of health states assessed, means and standard deviations should not be compared across scales, but they can be used as benchmarks for other studies. Appendix C provides the same information stratified by type of depression and clinician specialty, as well as means and standard deviations for *change* in HRQOL over two years.

One problem often encountered in measuring health outcomes is that scores cluster at the lowest or highest scores, that is, a "floor" or "ceiling" effect. When this occurs, the measure may not be precise enough to show health changes for those clustered at one end of the distribution. For most HRQOL measures, the full range of functioning is captured, but there is clustering at one extreme for six measures, although they are less skewed for depressed patients than for other populations (McHorney et al., 1994; Stewart and Ware, 1992). On some measures, severely depressed patients are more likely to have the worst possible score.[11]

The internal-consistency reliability coefficients for all measures exceed the usual rule of thumb for group comparisons (0.50) and sometimes even for individual comparisons (0.90) (Table 5.7 and Appendix C).[12]

We evaluated construct validity, or the extent to which correlations among HRQOL measures confirmed hypothesized patterns, and the extent to which measures were biased by socially desirable responding. The fourteen scales showed acceptable construct validity.[13] Different baseline measures *within* the global mental and physical health domains are more highly correlated with one another than with measures from the other global construct, supporting a model of two distinct but overlapping health domains. A two-domain pattern holds for patients with subthreshold depression, major depressive disorder alone, and dysthymia alone (see Appendix C), but a *single construct* solution is supported for patients with double depression, which means that studies of patients with double depression could include fewer HRQOL measures. The HRQOL measures had only very low correlations with a measure of socially desirable responding.[14]

Regarding concurrent validity (the relationship of HRQOL measures to clinical status at a point in time), the correlation between the depressive symptoms measure and each mental health-related HRQOL measure is in the same range (.50–.60) (see Table 5.8) as correlations among mental health HRQOL measures themselves; the correlations of depressive symptom counts with physical health HRQOL domains are lower, in the .20–.30 range.

Predictive validity was evaluated by comparing change in HRQOL and change in clinical status (Table 5.8, columns 2 and 3). Patients

Table 5.7 Characteristics of HRQOL Measures for Depressed Patients

Measure	No. of items	Mean	SD	Reliability	Item–total correlations	Floor (%)	Ceiling (%)	Complete data (%)
Physical functioning (+)[a]	10	72.3	27.9	.93	.53–.82	1	24	89
Serious limitations (−)	4	1.4	1.2	.73	.43–.71	29	7	—
Role–physical (+)	4	50.2	39.4	.85	.69–.73	26	29	94
Role–emotional (+)	3	46.6	40.5	.79	.57–.69	32	30	96
Bodily pain (+)	2	59.5	23.5	.78	.64	2	16	94
Mental health (+)	5	56.3	21.2	.88	.54–.79	<1	<1	92
Cognitive functioning (+)	6	73.1	18.7	.88	.60–.78	0	7	90
Social functioning (+)	2	67.8	27.3	.84	.73	2	24	95
Sexual functioning (−)	5	33.1	35.1	.89	.65–.83	35	9	89
Marital functioning (+)	6	62.1	23.3	.84	.38–.71	<1	4	85
Energy/fatigue (+)	4	45.6	21.1	.85	.66–.71	2	<1	94
Sleep problems (−)	6	36.8	19.7	.78	.41–.62	<1	<1	94
Physical/psychophysiologic symptoms (−)	7	29.3	18.5	.70	.34–.52	2	0	90
General health perceptions (+)	5	55.6	21.6	.76	.33–.72	<1	<1	92

Note: Floor = lowest possible score; ceiling = highest possible score.

a. A (+) high score indicates better health; a (−) high score indicates worse health.

Table 5.8 Correlations[a] between Current Symptoms and Functioning and Well-Being Measures and Point Changes in HRQOL over Two Years by Remission Status

	Current symptoms	Remitted	
		Yes	No
Physical functioning (+)[b]	−.16**	4.0	−0.1
Serious limitations (−)	.30**	−0.2	−0.1
Role–physical (+)	−.25**	14.7*	1.0
Role–emotional (+)	−.48**	26.0*	13.5
Bodily pain (+)	−.22**	5.1	1.8
Mental health (+)	−.61**	14.1**	5.5
Cognitive functioning (+)	−.53**	7.0	2.6
Social functioning (+)	−.50**	13.9**	4.2
Sexual functioning (−)	.21**	−8.6	−9.9
Marital functioning (+)	−.24**	7.3	1.3
Energy/fatigue (+)	−.36**	14.1*	8.4
Sleep problems (−)	.37**	−5.9	−5.2
Physical/psychophysiologic symptoms (−)	.24**	−3.4	−1.0
General health perceptions (+)	−.26**	10.8**	−0.6

*p < .05; **p < .01 or less.
a. Correlations between measures at the end of two years of the study.
b. A (+) high score indicates better health; a (−) high score indicates worse health.

who remitted had greater improvement in thirteen of fourteen domains of HRQOL than those who did not remit (six of them were statistically significant). This information can be used to help interpret HRQOL measures. For example, one can say that an eleven-point increase in general health perceptions in depressed patients is equivalent to the effect of remission of major depression.

Choosing Measures of Quality and Outcomes of Care

The MOS developed a rich framework to measure outcomes of care for depression and attempted a new strategy to measure process of clinical care. This set of measures may be too comprehensive or too expensive for most purposes. How, then, should one select among these measures?

Process of Care

For processes of clinical care, the most important measures are those with a known relationship with health outcomes or costs. Our short list of five straightforward measures covers the most common processes of care that would be expected to affect outcomes for depressed patients:

1. Detection, from the clinician post-visit form. Detection determines whether treatment occurs, even though it does not influence outcomes by itself.
2. Patient use of antidepressant medication (based on name, dosage, periods of use in last six months and any use in last month, cost), from patient report. Effective antidepressant medication is currently the most direct indicator of efficacious treatment.
3. Patient use of minor tranquilizers (same information as antidepressant medication, except that dosage is not needed), from patient report. Regular minor tranquilizer use addresses one *overuse* problem that is rarely examined in clinical trials but that has cost and possibly outcome implications.
4. Counseling for depression during a visit when the patient is acutely depressed, from clinician post-visit form.
5. Clinician preference for counseling depression. This style measure is less critical than counseling exposure (4) but holds promise for describing counseling in typical general practices because it predicts subsequent counseling behavior. Clinician-level style measures in general are not very reliable, however, and should not be used as a substitute for patient-level measures of quality of clinical treatments (measures 1–4) until further development and testing of these measures have been performed.

Health Outcomes

The outcome measures most central to the MOS research questions are domains of HRQOL. The functioning measures (serious limitations in physical and role functioning) seem to be particularly important because they directly reflect the societal burden of depression. Measures of psychological distress and well-being overlap with depressive symptoms and could be assessed through either the HRQOL or clinical assessment approach. Clinical outcomes are usually more expensive to measure, however, because they require a structured diagnostic instrument or clinician observation, although some self-report measures of depressive symptoms, such as the Center for Epidemiologic Studies Depression Scale, are available.

How many different measures of HRQOL outcomes are needed? In the context of busy clinical practices, very brief assessments are required. One strategy would be to begin with the SF-36 scales and the serious limitations measure. The serious limitations measure was more useful than the SF-36 scales in the MOS for evaluating care for depression, but this needs to be studied further before recommending it generally. This brief assessment can then be expanded with measures of cognitive functioning, sexual and marital functioning, sleep problems, and physical /psychological symptoms, depending on the goals of the particular evaluation. For evaluating treatments that focus on cognitive or sexual functioning, measures beyond the standard MOS short-form measures should be included.

Other Considerations and Future Developments

Policymakers want singular and integrative indicators of outcome that can provide guidance in resource allocation decisions. Many such decisions require choosing between interventions with very different characteristics, and multiple outcome comparisons generally yield confusing contradictions. A "bottom-line" measure that can be used in cost-effectiveness / utility analyses would be particularly relevant. Unfortunately, this is an area that needs more development. The SF-36 has global mental and physical functioning measures based on factor scores of the component scales (Sherbourne et al., 1995; Ware et al., 1994), but they require measurement of all scales and still do not provide a single overall number.

Utilities, or patient preferences for outcomes, is a concept that provides a uniform or common metric (the value of outcomes) for evaluating outcomes across different patient groups or health care systems. Most researchers would consider this the *theoretically* most appropriate measure to be used for cost-effectiveness analyses (Kamlet, 1992; Torrance, 1986). Some approaches to the assessment of HRQOL have developed utility weights (Kaplan et al., 1976; Kaplan and Anderson, 1988), but there remain many unresolved *practical* problems, including the best method of assessment and the validity of utilities. Important developments that could enable cost-utility analyses in the future would include validated algorithms to map self-reported functioning and well-being measures into utilities. At the moment, however, the best alternative may be to choose an outcome that appears to be relevant for a wide range of conditions. This is the approach we take in the cost-effectiveness analysis in Chapter 9.

There are several other areas for future improvements in assessing processes of care and outcomes. Clinicians distinguish acute-care from continuity and maintenance phases, but the MOS had no approach to analyze these distinct phases. Analyzing episodes of appropriate care based on clinical characteristics might be a promising approach. This approach could adapt ideas developed in utilization-based analyses of health care episodes (Keeler et al., 1988; Kessler et al., 1980).

The assessment of counseling and psychotherapy in usual care settings also requires more development to study how it differs from structured psychotherapies in clinical trials and to determine the efficacy of these applied and probably more heterogeneous forms of psychotherapy. Measures of counseling style are needed that capture cost differences (group versus individual therapy) and that identify specific counseling activities from the perspective of one or more efficacious forms of psychotherapy, such as cognitive or interpersonal psychotherapy. The relationship of measures of counseling to traditional utilization measures should also be explored. The issue goes well beyond measurement toward a new generation of psychotherapy-effectiveness studies.

In the area of health outcomes, the meaning of observed differences in HRQOL scales has not yet been adequately addressed. Although some information has been published to guide interpretation of differences in SF-36 scale scores (McHorney, Ware, and Raczek, 1993; Ware et al., 1994), more evaluation of score differences, such as scaling them against clinical changes, is needed for depression. A related issue that needs further study is whether differences in scale scores have a similar interpretation at different scale values or for different groups (for example, the young and the very old). Floor and ceiling effects in HRQOL measures can be important and may limit the assessment of the full impact of the condition for sicker patients on some scales. Scales with large floor or ceiling effects should be a high priority for refinement. In applications that require sensitivity to change over a very short time-frame, such as inpatient stays (days or weeks), it may be necessary to modify item content accordingly, but such changes need to be re-evaluated in terms of reliability and validity. Most important, however, may be some validation of the MOS measures to counter criticism that self-report is invalid because depressed patients incorrectly report their functioning as a result of negative cognitions that are part of the symptom complex of depression (Beck et al., 1962). This is not a trivial task, as methods of directly validating reports of functioning, such as independent observations, are very costly and can be biased or can cause Hawthorne effects (alter functioning of the observed patient).

Although these future efforts need to be made, the simple process of care and health outcomes measures recommended here will provide useful standards of comparison for studies whose goal is to describe the level of quality of care and health outcomes for depressed outpatients.

Chapter Six

Social and Clinical Factors

In this chapter we discuss how depression compares with common medical conditions, such as hypertension, diabetes, arthritis, and heart disease, and how depressed patients are distributed across health care delivery systems. We address three questions:

1. How common is depression in typical general medical practices and mental health specialty practices compared with medical conditions?
2. How limited are depressed patients in their daily functioning and well-being, and how do they compare with patients with medical conditions?
3. How are depressed patients distributed across payment systems or specialty sectors, and how does patient sickness differ?

The answers to the first two questions show why depression is socially and clinically important and why care for depression should be evaluated. The answer to the third question indicates which delivery systems need to anticipate higher burdens on resources in terms of patient needs. This is also important for making meaningful comparisons of care for depression across delivery settings because patient groups that differ in health status are likely to differ in treatments, costs, and health outcomes.

Prevalence of Depression

Subthreshold depression in the MOS was defined as exceeding the screener but not having a current disorder. The prevalence of subthreshold depression is therefore the probability of exceeding the screener, weighted for sampling design and nonresponse, excluding patients with current disorder. To estimate the prevalence of depressive disorder we used a two-part model reflecting the two-stage casefinding. The first step estimates the probability of exceeding the depression screener cut-point; the second step is the probability of meeting criteria for current unipolar depressive disorder, conditional on exceeding the screener cut-point. The product of these two probabilities for any practice setting represents the estimated prevalence of depressive disorder among all practice patients in that setting, after correcting for the estimated sensitivity of the first-stage screener in that practice setting. This correction is necessary because the screener does not detect all patients with depressive disorder.[1]

Figure 6.1 shows the estimated prevalence of depressive disorder and symptoms in different MOS practice settings. Across systems of care, 7 percent of general medical patients and 32 percent of mental health specialty patients were estimated to have current depressive disorder (major depression or dysthymia) and about 25 percent of general medical patients and 63 percent of mental health specialty patients exceeded the cut-point on the first-stage depression screener, meaning that they had at least two weeks or more of feeling sad in the prior year and were likely to have current symptoms. Prevalence

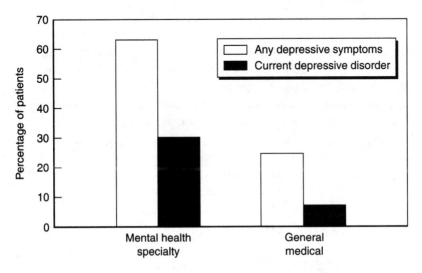

Figure 6.1   Prevalence of Depressive Symptoms and Disorder by Specialty

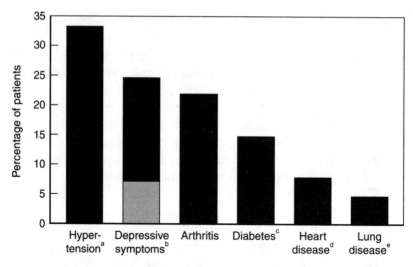

a. High blood pressure.
b. Any depressive symptoms; light shade is current depressive disorder.
c. High blood sugar or diabetes.
d. Heart attack (lifetime) or current heart failure or enlarged heart.
e. Asthma or other severe lung problems such as chronic bronchitis or
   emphysema.

Figure 6.2   Prevalence of Depression and Patient-Reported Medical Conditions,
General Medical Practices

differs significantly by specialty but not by type of payment (PP or
FFS), both within and across specialty sectors.[2]

Figure 6.2 shows that depression (current disorder or subthreshold)
was as prevalent as the most common chronic medical conditions in
general medical practices, affecting about 25 percent of these outpatients, making it second only to hypertension. Seven percent had
depressive disorder, quite similar to serious heart disease (defined as
ever having a heart attack or current congestive heart failure). Based
on prevalence alone, depression appears to be an important clinical
condition across health care systems. Whether this should translate
into equivalent attention by providers, employers, and policymakers
depends in part on how strongly depression affects individuals.

How Depression Affects Functioning and Well-Being

A broad perspective of health, including physical functioning, bodily
pain, role functioning, and the other domains of health discussed in

Chapter 5, informs policy decisions about the allocation of services and insurance coverage as it allows comparisons across different disease conditions. One problem, however, is the difficulty of proving that one specific disease condition causes morbidity, because other injuries or concurrent disease conditions might be responsible. Experimental trials are of little help—although one can assign sick individuals to different treatments, one cannot assign healthy individuals to different diseases. In the MOS, two approaches were used to estimate the association of depression and morbidity, a cross-sectional and a longitudinal approach.

Cross-sectional approach. We first used cross-sectional data and multiple regression methods to estimate the level of morbidity that patients with a specific condition have after accounting for all their other conditions. The covariates included patient demographics, system-of-care effects, and the other medical conditions present. We call the effect that is attributed to depression after we take out the effect of other disease conditions "depression's unique association" with morbidity.[3]

Figure 6.3 provides a striking scorecard of depression's unique association with functioning. Depression in this scorecard includes depressive disorder and depressive symptoms only. The columns represent six domains of functioning and well-being from Table 5.6. For each medical condition (represented by rows), the box indicates how the condition compares with depression on morbidity: a black box means that depressed patients have significantly greater morbidity; a gray box indicates no significant difference in morbidity; and a white box indicates that the medical condition has greater morbidity.

For most domains of functioning, depression is more debilitating than most medical conditions. Only serious heart disease (myocardial infarction in the prior year or current congestive heart failure) and arthritis are associated with greater morbidity in any domain of functioning. Serious heart disease imposes greater physical and role limitations and more bed days, and arthritis is associated with more bodily pain.

Figure 6.4 provides a closer look at one measure of morbidity—the number of days per month spent entirely in bed. Only serious heart disease is associated with more bed days (2 in a month rather than 1.5). But because depressive symptoms are much more prevalent than heart disease, depression accounts for a larger number of bed days among all outpatients.

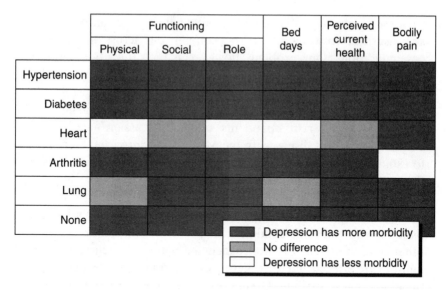

	Functioning			Bed days	Perceived current health	Bodily pain
	Physical	Social	Role			
Hypertension						
Diabetes						
Heart						
Arthritis						
Lung						
None						

■ Depression has more morbidity
▨ No difference
□ Depression has less morbidity

Figure 6.3 Depression Morbidity "Scorecard": Comparison with Chronic Medical Conditions

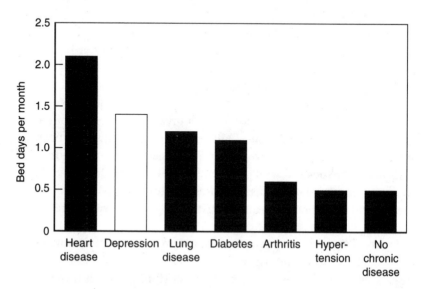

Figure 6.4 Bed Days Associated with Depression or Other Disease Conditions Alone

Longitudinal approach. Depression is often episodic or involves only a single episode, whereas the medical conditions studied in the MOS are chronic and can have a progressively deteriorating clinical course, although remissions are possible. This could mean that depression has less of an impact over time than a chronic medical condition.

Hays et al. (1995) compared change in functioning over time on each domain for patients with each type of depression (depression symptoms only and each current disorder group) in the general medical and mental health specialty sectors, and for general medical patients with each of several chronic medical conditions.[4] Depressed patients tended to improve over time, whereas persons with chronic medical conditions tended to stay the same or get worse in physical morbidity. Nevertheless, depressed patients continued to have equivalent or even worse functioning and well-being than medical patients at the second year of follow-up. Depressed patients improved primarily in general health perceptions and in the psychological domains of emotional well-being, role-emotional functioning, social functioning, and energy / fatigue, but not in the physical functioning domains.

Figure 6.5 shows baseline and two-year levels of physical functioning and social functioning for general medical patients with double depression or early-onset diabetes at baseline. In each domain, the patients with double depression improved, especially in social functioning. Despite deteriorating health, diabetics had *less* morbidity at two years than double-depressed patients. Similarly, the absolute level of functioning or well-being for all depressed general medical patients and for depressed mental health specialty patients was comparable to or worse than it was for patients with chronic medical conditions after two years.

Patients with subthreshold depression remained essentially unchanged in functioning and well-being over the two years, and their limitations remained in the range of morbidity of medical patients. Thus subthreshold depressive symptoms were not a transient condition, but one of persistent and substantial morbidity.

One possible explanation for this finding is that subthreshold depression is a variant of affective disorder. If subthreshold depressive symptoms primarily represent another form of affective disorder, patients with such symptoms should be more similar to patients with

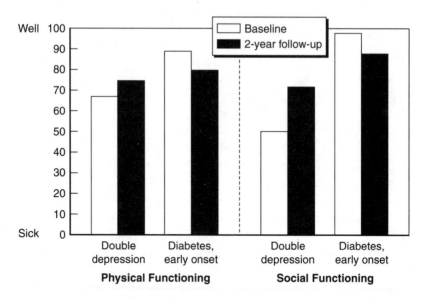

Figure 6.5   Depressed Patients Improve but Remain Limited (General Medical
Practices)

depressive disorder than to nondepressed patients in demographics
and other clinical features (such as extent of psychiatric and medical
comorbidities). We tested these hypotheses by comparing patients
with subthreshold depression versus affective disorder within and
across specialty sectors; and within the general medical sector, by
comparing hypertensive patients without depression with those who
had subthreshold symptoms or depressive disorder.[5]

Patients with subthreshold depression and depressive disorder
were similar in demographic characteristics and comorbidities, except
that patients with depressive disorder had a much higher prevalence
of generalized anxiety (62 percent compared with 31 percent for
subthreshold depression) and panic disorder (20 percent compared
with 4 percent, respectively). The two depression groups were more
similar in the mental health specialty than the general medical sector.
Among patients with subthreshold symptoms, 41 percent had at least
one first-degree relative with a history of depression. Although this
was significantly less than the 59 percent with current depressive
disorder, it is a surprisingly high rate, suggesting that subthreshold
symptoms could be a variant of primary affective disorder.

The Distribution of Depressed Patients across Practice Settings

Most depressed patients receive care in general medicine, not in mental health specialty, regardless of payment system. This does not necessarily mean that patients are being treated for their depression, as the MOS identified depressed patients independently from their providers. Figure 6.6 shows the distribution of patients across specialty sectors by payment structure for the panel of patients with any depressive symptoms.[6] Under PP care, the percentage of patients visiting a general medical provider was slightly higher; the percentage of patients visiting psychologists or master's-level therapists was significantly higher; and the percentage visiting psychiatrists was significantly lower (about half the percentage in FFS). Controlling for patient demographics and baseline psychological and physical sickness does not change the conclusions.[7]

We also tested whether payment systems differed in targeting sick patients to specialty care. In both payment systems, patients' health status was one of the most influential factors determining which provider specialty they visited. Worse psychological health increased

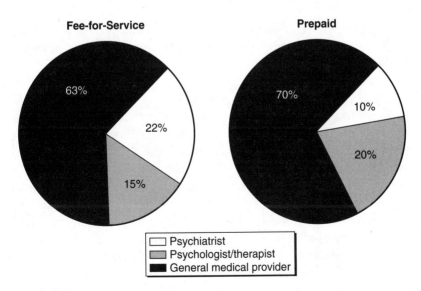

Figure 6.6 Who Treats Depressed Patients, by Payment Type (Percentage of Patients Treated by Each Specialty Sector)

the probability of obtaining care from a mental health specialist, and worse physical health increased the probability of obtaining care from a general medical provider, but there was no difference between PP and FFS in this relationship. The results indicated that *both* payment systems tended to target psychologically sicker patients to mental health specialty care, in contrast with earlier studies which found that there is no targeting (Cooper-Patrick, Crum, and Ford, 1994; Frank and Kamlet, 1989).[8]

Establishing whether or not there are differences in casemix and how great these differences are is critical to process and outcome comparisons in a nonexperimental study. It is also of direct clinical and educational interest because it informs whether similar treatments are indicated for different patient groups. We therefore studied casemix differences in more detail. Overall, there are no differences by payment types, making direct quality-of-care comparisons unproblematic. There are significant differences across provider specialty, however, necessitating that quality-of-care comparisons pay attention to selection bias.

Mental Health Status

We first compared severity of depression across provider specialty and payment by focusing on patients with current depressive disorder, as this is the group most often used for clinical studies.[9]

Patients of psychiatrists tended to be the most psychologically sick, and patients of general medical clinicians the least psychologically sick across a variety of measures of severity of depression or psychopathology. As shown in Figure 6.7, the Hamilton Depression Rating Scale score (a common measure of severity in clinical trials) averaged twenty for patients of psychiatrists and only sixteen for patients of other provider groups. Patients of psychiatrists had also experienced more symptoms of depression in their lifetime (twenty compared with sixteen to twenty) and were more likely to have had double depression than patients of other specialty sectors. Patients of psychologists and master's-level therapists generally had an intermediate level of severity of depression, between that of patients of psychiatrists and that of general medical providers. Patients of both psychiatrists and other mental health specialists were more

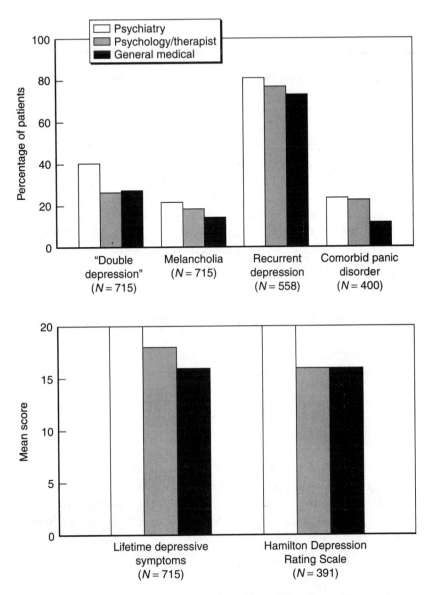

Figure 6.7   Mental Health Specialty Patients Have More Severe Depression

likely to have melancholia, a severe form of depression in terms of symptomatic presentation, than patients in the general medical sector.

Patients with recurrent depression (two or more prior spells of depression) were at high risk for future episodes and benefited from maintenance therapy, such as long-run antidepressant medication. The rate of recurrent depression was highest in psychiatry, although the majority of patients in all specialty sectors had recurrent depression. These specialty differences in casemix are large, systematically in the same direction (psychiatrists have the psychologically sickest patients), and robust to adjusting for multiple statistical comparisons. One reason we find significant differences, whereas earlier studies from the ECA (Cooper-Patrick, Crum, and Ford, 1994; Frank and Kamlet, 1989) did not, may simply be that we had a larger sample size of depressed patients, and therefore better statistical power to detect differences.[10]

In contrast, there is no substantial evidence that sickness systematically differs by payment system. Some payment or specialty-payment interactions are significant, but differences are not in the same direction and probably reflect random variation: at a 5 percent level of significance, one expects that one out of twenty tests is significant even if there is no underlying difference.

Comorbidity

Comorbidities, whether psychiatric or medical, complicate depression treatment (Popkin, Callies, and MacKenzie, 1985; Rodin, Craven, and Littlefield, 1991). We analyzed comorbid chronic medical conditions, anxiety disorder, and alcoholism for the sample with lifetime depressive disorder.[11]

Chronic Medical Conditions

Two-thirds of patients had at least one comorbid major chronic medical condition (Figure 6.8), and those patients averaged two chronic conditions. This finding casts doubts on the generalizability of the efficacy results of clinical trials for typical depressed patients because clinical trials often exclude patients on the basis of comorbidities.

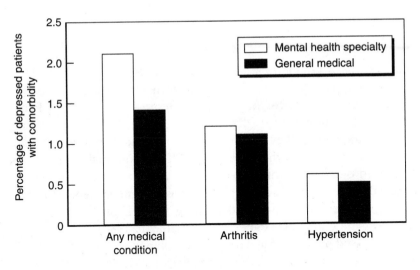

Figure 6.8 Medical Comorbidity by Specialty

Such trials have atypical depressed samples and do not provide appropriate guidance for care of the majority of depressed patients in private practice settings.

Although the prevalence of *any* medical comorbidity did not differ by payment or specialty, hypertension and arthritis were significantly more common among depressed patients of general medical clinicians than among patients of mental health specialists. Moreover, the general medical sector had more severe cases: among patients with hypertension, 55 percent in general medical practices used an antihypertensive medication at the screening visit, compared with only 37 percent in mental health specialty; among patients reporting diabetes, 14 percent in general medical practices took insulin injections, compared with only 2 percent in mental health specialty. There were no differences by specialty in prevalence of diabetes, gastrointestinal disorder, chronic lung disease, back problems, or advanced heart disease, suggesting that the mental health specialty sector as well as the general medical sector should be equally prepared to treat patients in the context of comorbid medical conditions.[12] In contrast with provider specialty, we found no significant differences in any measure of chronic medical comorbidity by payment system.

Psychiatric Conditions

We also considered two psychiatric comorbid conditions common in the depressed population: anxiety disorder and alcoholism.[13] Alcoholism is especially critical because it must often be treated before depression can be successfully treated (Depression Guidelines Panel, 1993), and it may increase depression or further limit depressed patients' functioning. Any differences in comorbid alcoholism by payment type or specialty therefore imply different optimal treatments or expected outcomes. Similarly, comorbid anxiety disorder, especially panic disorder, requires determining which is primary (earlier onset), and some experts recommend treating the primary condition first (Depression Guidelines Panel, 1993a; Schuckit, 1986).

Depressed patients of general medical clinicians had a significantly lower rate of panic disorder (11 percent) and one-year alcohol disorder (5 percent) than patients of psychiatrists or other mental health specialists (22–23 percent for panic disorder, 13 percent for alcoholism). Recent problems related to drinking or the amount of alcohol recently consumed did not differ by specialty, but patients of mental health specialists were almost twice as likely to say they needed help for alcoholism or another drug problem (14 percent versus 8 percent).

Regarding payment systems, 17 percent of FFS mental health specialty patients had comorbid current alcohol disorder, compared with 4–9 percent across other specialty-payment groups (Figure 6.9), but there were no differences in comorbid panic disorder.

Functioning and Well-Being

Functioning and well-being integrate severity differences across various conditions because they are not disease-specific. The baseline differences by specialty and payment generally parallel clinical casemix.[14]

Mental health specialty depressed patients were sicker in psychosocial domains, whereas general medical patients were sicker in the somatic domains of health. Among physical health domains, patients of general medical providers were significantly sicker than patients of mental health specialists in physical functioning, pain, and general health perceptions, but not in role-physical functioning. Among mental health domains, mental health specialty patients had somewhat

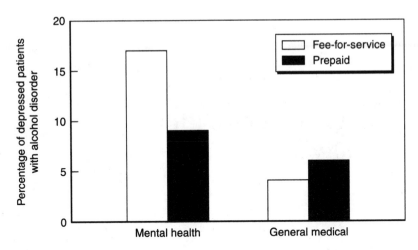

Figure 6.9   Fee-for-Service Mental Health Specialty Patients Have More Current Alcohol Disorder

worse scores in overall mental health status and limitations in social activities, but the differences were not significant for cognitive functioning or role-emotional functioning. There were no significant differences by specialty in a third set of domains that represents overlapping physical and mental health constructs (symptoms, energy / fatigue, health distress, and sleep problems). Clearly, morbidity differences reflect clinical sickness differences: once one controls for medical comorbidity, the significant difference in bodily pain disappears. Similarly, the difference in social activities disappeared when we controlled for depression severity in regression analyses.

All differences in morbidity were by provider specialty; there were no systematic differences by type of payment or interactions between specialty and type of payment.[15]

Chapter Seven

How Treatment Differs by Specialty and Payment

In this chapter we compare quality of care and utilization of services across payment systems and specialty sectors for depressed patients by analyzing the components introduced in Chapter 5: detection, psychotropic medication, counseling, utilization, and continuity of care. Overall, there is an obvious gap between what one would assume about treatment of depressed patients based on the more widely available clinical efficacy studies and recommendations in clinical practice guidelines and standard clinical textbooks, and what patients actually receive in typical settings. Documenting this gap is an important component of education efforts and quality-assurance programs.

Detection

The efficacy of treatment is well established for patients with depressive disorder, but not for patients with subthreshold depressive symptoms (Depression Guidelines Panel, 1993b). We therefore limit this analysis to patients with current disorder, where failure to detect is unambiguously an indication of poor quality of care.

We obtained detection information at the end of the original visit by asking clinicians if the patient had a clinically meaningful depression for two weeks or more any time in the past year. As Figure 7.1 indicates, patients visiting general medical clinicians had little more than a 50 percent chance of having their current depressive disorder detected, and those receiving PP care had even lower rates of detec-

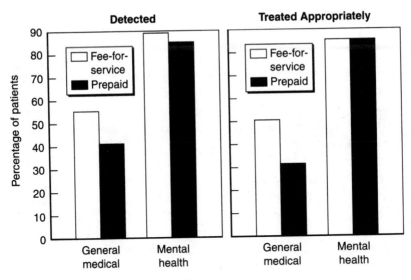

Figure 7.1   Detection and Appropriate Treatment of Current Depressive Disorder Lower in General Medical Care

tion than those in FFS care. General medical clinicians were much less likely than mental health specialists to detect and treat depression, even after controlling for differences in level of depressive symptoms, general health status, patient demographics, duration of visit, and recency of last health care visit to minimize casemix biases. Thus lower rates of detection in general medicine and PP care are due not simply to shorter visits or less frequent visits, but to other aspects of the treatment environment, such as incentives to reduce services or referral rates or differences in attitudes toward treating depression.

We reach the same conclusion when considering the percentage of patients receiving "appropriate treatment"—here defined as having depression detected and treated in the visit through either counseling or referral by the MOS clinician or awareness by the clinician that another provider was treating the depression. The rate of overall appropriate care was much higher for mental health specialists, regardless of payment type.[1] When the same analyses were repeated for different practice organizations (HMOs, MSGs, and SOLOs), there were no significant differences by organization, because the PP and FFS patients in MSGs and SOLOs were combined, counterbalancing the payment-related differences.

Psychotropic Medication

We focus on two broad groups of psychotropic medication, antidepressants and minor tranquilizers, which account for most psychotropic medications prescribed. Because of the strong evidence for the efficacy of antidepressant medications (Depression Guidelines Panel, 1993b), differences in their use have direct implications for the effectiveness of overall care. In contrast, there is little evidence that minor tranquilizers are efficacious for depression; they could even be interpreted as overused because they are costly and have side effects, including risk for addiction with long-term use. Minor tranquilizers can be appropriately prescribed for a reason other than depression, however, including for comorbid anxiety disorder or during the latency phase of antidepressant medication effects.

About 59 percent of depressed patients in the MOS used neither an antidepressant nor a minor tranquilizer; 12 percent used only an antidepressant; 19 percent used only a minor tranquilizer; and 11 percent used both. "Use" means having used the medication in the prior month or having used it daily for a month or more in the prior six months. The results therefore primarily refer to regular use (at least a month) of psychotropic medications.[2]

Figure 7.2 shows the use of psychotropic medications by specialty at baseline, stratified by patient sickness (here displayed through the highest and lowest quartiles of the global psychological sickness scale) and adjusted for other differences in patient sickness and demographic characteristics. Psychiatrists were most likely to prescribe antidepressant medications and minor tranquilizers at each level of psychological sickness. Because we control for casemix, we know that the higher rate of medication, including minor tranquilizers, among psychiatry patients is not due to their greater level of psychological sickness. About half of patients of psychiatrists with high severity and just under a third of those with low severity used an antidepressant medication. Given that the high-severity patients virtually all had current disorder plus high levels of depressive symptoms, it may be surprising that half of these patients of psychiatrists were not using antidepressant medications.

The average percentage of patients using antidepressant medications was similarly low for psychologists and master's-level therapists and general medical clinicians. As shown in Figure 7.2, however, there

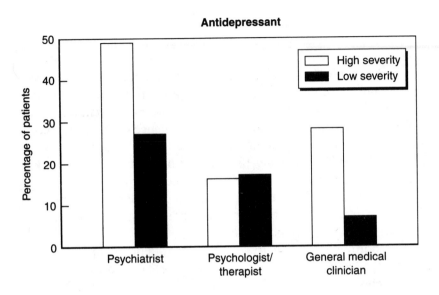

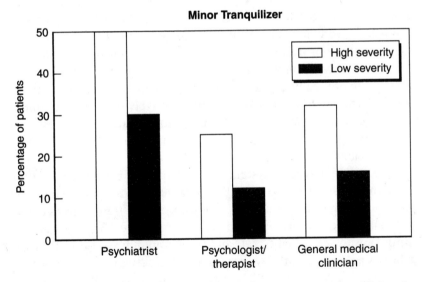

Figure 7.2 Psychotropic Medication Use Is Only Moderate, but Higher for Psychiatric Patients (Data drawn from *American Journal of Psychiatry*, May 1994 [151:5]. Copyright 1994, the American Psychiatric Association. Reprinted by permission.)

was a different response to the level of psychological sickness by specialty. The sicker patients of general medical clinicians and psychiatrists were more likely to use antidepressants (that is, about a doubling in percentage using antidepressant medication for those in the highest and lowest quartile on the global psychological sickness scale). In contrast, for patients of nonphysicians (psychologists and master's-level therapists), there was no evidence of any difference in medication use corresponding to sickness level. As the nonphysician therapist is not prescribing the medication, this suggests a lack of coordination between the nonphysician therapist and the prescribing physician, a predominant psychosocial theoretical and treatment orientation, or insufficient training in the indications for antidepressant medication among nonphysicians.

The bottom half of Figure 7.2 shows that depressed patients were at least as likely to use minor tranquilizers as antidepressant medications. This is true across all sickness levels; minor tranquilizers were not reserved just for less sick patients, nor were antidepressant medications exclusively used by sicker patients. The sicker patients of physicians were most likely to receive both types of medications. Given that minor tranquilizers are not considered first-line treatment for severe depression and that use of multiple psychotropic medications is theoretically a strategy reserved for the minority of patients who are treatment nonresponders, the relatively high levels of minor tranquilizer use and combined medication treatment suggest that basic principles of clinical practice guidelines are not being followed by physicians.

At baseline, payment systems did not differ in prior use of antidepressants after adjusting for patient characteristics. PP patients were more likely than FFS patients to be using minor tranquilizers across specialties and within each specialty sector (Figure 7.3), however. It is surprising to see a higher rate of minor tranquilizer use in PP care, which is associated with lower rates of use of services and is presumed to reduce inefficient use. This difference in use cannot be explained by casemix, as there was no significant difference between FFS and PP patients in average symptoms of anxiety, prevalence of panic disorder, comorbid alcoholism, or use of alprazolam (for which there is some efficacy evidence in depression). These results are weighted for sampling probability and nonresponse and the qualitative results are robust, although unweighted differences are smaller. Across all

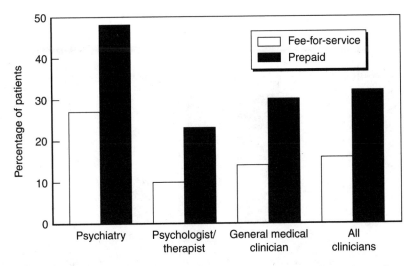

Figure 7.3　Minor Tranquilizer Use Is Higher in Prepaid Care (Data drawn from *American Journal of Psychiatry*, May 1994 [151:5]. Copyright 1994, the American Psychiatric Association. Reprinted by permission.)

MOS tracer conditions, prepayment was not associated with high rates of minor tranquilizer use except among depressed patients, making this a specific quality problem for this condition.

We evaluated effective antidepressant medications by requiring minimum therapeutic dosage levels (Depression Guidelines Panel, 1993b; Katon et al., 1992). These minimum levels were very low, equivalent to 75 mg of imipramine daily for the nonelderly and 50 mg daily for the elderly. Among the 144 patients using any antidepressant medication, 56 (39 percent) used a subtherapeutic daily dosage. At baseline, this percentage did not vary by payment or clinician specialty.

We also considered the duration of antidepressant medication, which is important because the majority of the depressed patients in the MOS sample had recurrent depression and could have benefited from long-run maintenance therapy (Depression Panel Guidelines, 1993b). PP patients of psychiatrists were more likely to discontinue antidepressant medication earlier than FFS patients of psychiatrists (Figure 7.4). For patients of general medical clinicians and for those of other mental health specialists, the level of decline in use of an effective antidepressant medication was similar in PP and FFS. This finding is clinically important, because psychiatrists had the most severely depressed patients, who have a high preva-

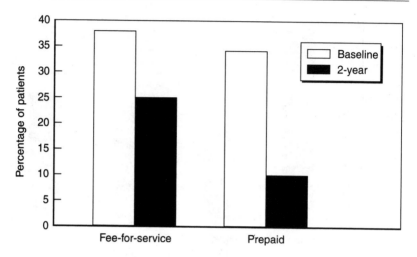

Figure 7.4   Use of Effective Antidepressant Medication Declines More Quickly in Prepaid Care for Patients of Psychiatrists

lence of recurrent depression and would therefore be candidates for maintenance therapy.

In sum, there were several problems with psychotropic medication management:

- relatively low rates of appropriate use, even by the sickest patients
- frequent use of multiple types of medication, a clinical strategy not generally recommended
- minor tranquilizers more commonly used than antidepressants as a first-line medication for depression
- early discontinuation of antidepressant medication in some practice settings

Counseling and Interpersonal Style of Care

Psychotherapy is the other commonly used efficacious treatment for depression in outpatients. We studied it using a provider-reported indicator of whether or not at least brief counseling (of three minutes or more) occurred during the screening visit (when the patient was acutely depressed and presumably might benefit from at least brief counseling). This is a better measure than it appears because the initial counseling visit is significantly associated with an additional eleven mental health visits during the first year for the most severely depressed patients, suggesting that a counseling visit indicates a more intensive course of treatment. In addition, we used provider-reported counseling style and depression treatment preferences across all patients (that is, not specific to the particular patients in the MOS patient panel), as well as general interpersonal style of care (not unique to depressed patients) to describe counseling style. These concepts are defined in Table 5.2.

Among patients with current depressive disorder at baseline, those visiting general medical providers were less likely than those visiting mental health specialists to be counseled for depression during the screening visit (Figure 7.5). In addition, patients of general medical providers were less likely to be counseled under PP than under FFS care.[3]

We also examined differences by payment in the therapy modality (individual, group, family, or other form of therapy). Most patients of mental health specialists received individual therapy (79 percent); 5 percent received group therapy; 5 percent received family therapy; 1 percent received other therapy; and 10 percent reported receiving no therapy. The distribution did differ significantly by payment, but most of the group therapy patients had less severe forms of depression (subthreshold depressive symptoms) and were PP patients. But re-

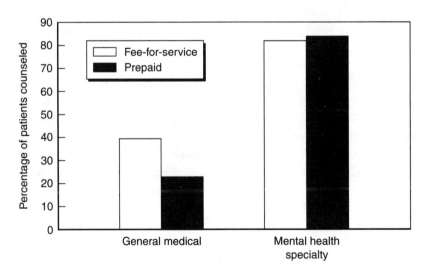

Figure 7.5   General Medical Patients with Depressive Disorder Are Less Likely to Be Counseled for Depression

gardless of payment type, the predominant mental health specialty therapy modality remains individual counseling.

Referral to mental health specialists was rarely used as an alternative to personal counseling in the general medical sector. Regardless of payment type, only 5–10 percent of general medical patients with depressive symptoms were referred to a mental health specialist at the time of the screening visit (Rogers et al., 1993).

The clinician-reported usual counseling style and interpersonal style of care differed primarily by specialty, less so by payment system, after adjusting for clinician demographic characteristics. Specialty comparisons were limited to general medical clinicians, psychiatrists, and psychologists (there were too few master's-level therapists for a clinician-level analysis). For the payment comparisons, clinicians were divided into those with fewer than 50 percent of patients under PP care, and those with 50 percent or more of their patients under PP care. The overall pattern of conclusions about these aspects of clinician style is summarized in Table 7.1.

Figure 7.6 shows the differences by specialty. There were no marked or significant differences by specialty in the level of aggressiveness, or initiative taken, in counseling. As expected, mental health specialists perceived themselves to be better skilled in counseling for personal problems and were more likely to provide face-to-face counseling. In addition, 75–81 percent of mental health specialists usually counseled for ten minutes or longer, compared with only 36 percent of general medical clinicians. Psychologists were the most likely to report that they usually counseled for ten minutes or more.

For counseling techniques, all specialty sectors typically relied on advice and education when counseling, but general medical clinicians relied significantly more on this technique. Mental health specialists, by contrast, relied much more than general medical clinicians on interpretation and confrontation and on formal psychodynamic therapy. Psychologists were especially likely to use behavioral therapy (69 percent) compared with psychiatrists (36 percent) or general medical clinicians (33 percent). Surprisingly, according to this self-report, psychiatrists were not more likely to use behavioral therapy than general medical clinicians. Compared with general medical providers, mental health specialists, especially psychiatrists, were more inclined to treat depression themselves rather than refer out. Overall, all specialists had a similar level of egalitarianism, in terms of attempting to use

Table 7.1   Summary of Specialty and Payment Differences in Counseling and Interpersonal Style of Care

Measure	Specialty difference (mental health specialty versus general medical)	Payment difference (more versus less of practice is prepaid)
Counseling style		
Initiative	No difference	No difference
Perceived skill	Mental health specialty: more skilled	No difference
Preference for depression counseling	Mental health specialty: stronger preference for counseling depressed patients	If more prepaid, less likely to counsel depressed patients
Intensity (duration)	Mental health specialty: more likely to have long sessions	If more prepaid patients, more likely to have short sessions
Technique	Mental health specialty: more psychodynamic therapy, more behavioral therapy (psychology); General medical: more advice/education	If more prepaid patients, more advice-oriented
Interpersonal style		
Egalitarian participation	No difference	No difference
Share treatment decision-making	Mental health specialty: more likely to share decisions with patients	No difference

their authority to influence patients. But mental health specialists were more oriented to sharing treatment decisions.

This pattern of differences in usual clinician treatment style makes sense intuitively. Psychiatrists are the most psychodynamically oriented, psychologists the most behaviorally oriented, but also psy-

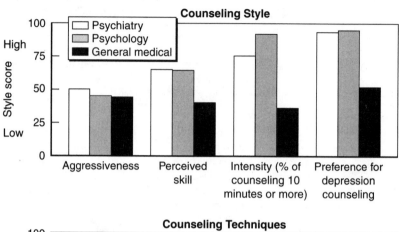

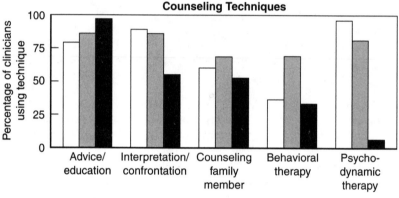

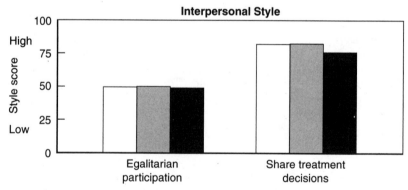

Figure 7.6 Specialty Differences in Clinician Usual Counseling and Interpersonal Style of Care

chodynamically oriented, and general medical clinicians primarily provide education and advice. At the same time, mental health specialists take more time when counseling, but not necessarily more initiative, than general medical clinicians. Mental health specialists report the highest level of skill in psychosocial counseling and a higher tendency than general medical providers to counsel personally rather than refer out. Mental health specialists are also more apt to share decisions with their patients.

There were only small payment differences. Clinicians with 50 percent or more PP patients reported a lower proclivity to counsel patients personally, were more likely to have counseling sessions under ten minutes in duration, and were more likely (96 percent versus 87 percent) to rely on education or advice when counseling. But there were no differences in interpersonal style of care. The results suggest that clinicians with more PP patients were somewhat more oriented toward brief, "reality-oriented" or advice-oriented therapy.

Plan Choice, Utilization, and Continuity of Care

Psychotropic medication and counseling or interpersonal style are direct indicators of processes of care related to quality of care, whereas utilization is a main cost component. From a policy perspective, we are particularly interested in whether PP care is associated with lower utilization rates, and whether this is related to quality of care or patient outcomes.

The first issue we address is the choice of payment plans. Switches between payment systems could substantially alter our conclusions about costs if high or low users tend to prefer one type of payment system to the other. Most previous studies assumed that such adverse selection would be related to health status, but this does not need to be the case. Individuals could simply differ systematically in their preferences for particular types of care or intensity of care.[4]

We found that about 11 percent of depressed patients switched financing plans in a year—a high rate for people with this level of sickness, considering that the literature suggests that sick patients with an established provider relationship are unlikely to switch. Although there was no *overall* significant net flow of patients from one payment system to the other, there was a significant difference in switching as a function of both provider specialty and payment system (an interaction effect): patients of mental health specialists were unlikely to switch out of FFS and much more likely to switch out of PP, whereas patients of general medical providers were very likely to switch out of FFS and much less likely to switch out of PP. This implies a net flow of patients to FFS mental health specialists and a net flow of patients to PP general medical providers. Selection by provider specialty could have major cost implications because the costs and utilization for patients receiving outpatient care from mental health specialists are substantially higher than for patients receiving general medical mental health care in prior experimental and observational studies (Frank and Kamlet, 1990; Wells et al., 1987).

Switching is an issue not only for the competitiveness of health plans, but also for the patient's health, especially for populations like the one represented by our sample, because switching to a new health care setting requires finding a new provider and establishing a new relationship. In the meantime, a patient may be without a source of care, a discontinuity that could lead to poorer outcomes. In the MOS, plan switching appeared to be related to an immediate decline in utilization for depressed patients, which was not followed by an increase or "catch-up" effect. The absence of the commonly found catch-up effect following switching and the significant decrease in utilization during the switching period suggested an interruption in care that did not occur for patients staying within a payment system. This finding emphasizes the need for integrating new patients quickly into a system, an issue that should not be neglected in the current policy discussion.

Our analysis of utilization focused on mental health outpatient visits, regardless of provider specialty.[5] Despite all the attention given to cost-offset effects, we found no evidence that patients with higher mental health utilization or specialty care or more appropriate care have reduced physical outpatient utilization or inpatient utilization. During the course of the study, probabilities of use of mental health services in a year were similar for FFS and PP and declined over time for each specialty sector (Figure 7.7). Among patients with at least one mental health visit, however, the average number of mental health visits was much lower in PP care; for example, there were 4.6 fewer visits in the six-month period before baseline, averaged across specialty sectors. The differences in level of use of mental health visits by payment were largely attributable to patients of psychiatrists and

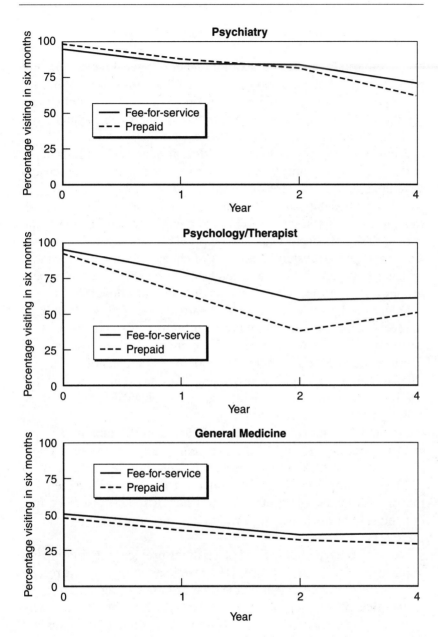

Figure 7.7   Percentage of Depressed Patients with a Mental Health Visit in the Last Six Months

persisted over time: even by the end of year two, patients initially treated by psychiatrists in PP had half the visits of those in FFS (eighteen versus nine in a six-month period; see Figure 7.8). For patients of psychologists and nonphysician therapists, use differences by payment were in the same direction but were not statistically significant. There was hardly any difference between payment systems in utilization in the general medical sector.

Provider continuity addresses a different dimension of utilization. It may also be a quality-of-care measure, but it was not sufficiently developed in the MOS for this purpose. Disruptions in the clinician-patient relationship could be due to plan-switching behavior, although the correlation between switching payment systems and ending the relationship with a given provider was surprisingly small. Thus there are a substantial number of changes in providers without switches between plans, and a significant number of patients appear to follow their providers across payment plans ("rollovers").[6]

Figure 7.9 shows the percentage of patients over time who continue to receive care from the initial provider by specialty and payment. In both payment systems, patients of nonphysician therapists (middle figure) ended the relationship earlier than did patients of either psychiatrists or general medical providers. This may reflect the fact that psychologists sometimes provide only psychological testing and assessment and not ongoing treatment.

Provider continuity was significantly lower in PP than in FFS psychiatric care. By the end of the two-year follow-up, the probability of continuing with the same psychiatrist was only .46 in PP, but .74 in FFS. PP patients changed providers earlier than FFS patients in the general medical and other mental health specialty sectors, too, but the difference between payment systems was not significant in these sectors.

We explored whether the end of a patient-provider relationship has implications for quality of care. When we focused on patients receiving effective antidepressant medication at baseline, the end of a patient-provider relationship was unambiguously associated with discontinuing antidepressant medication. Unfortunately, it was not possible to determine whether this occurred because patients no longer needed care or whether the relationship ended for some other reason and interrupted a beneficial medication therapy (but most patients in this sample had recurrent depression and would benefit

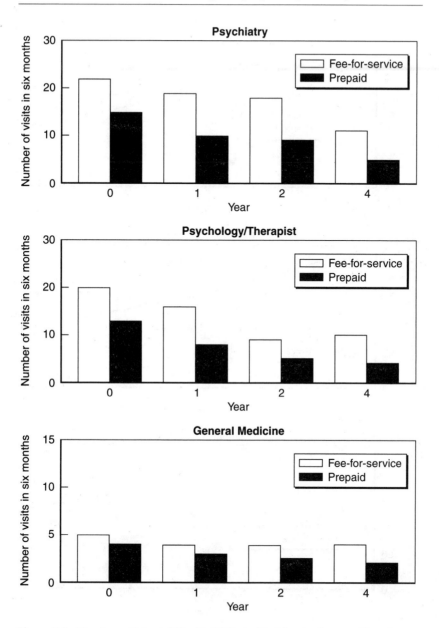

Figure 7.8   Number of Mental Health Visits in Six Months (among Users)

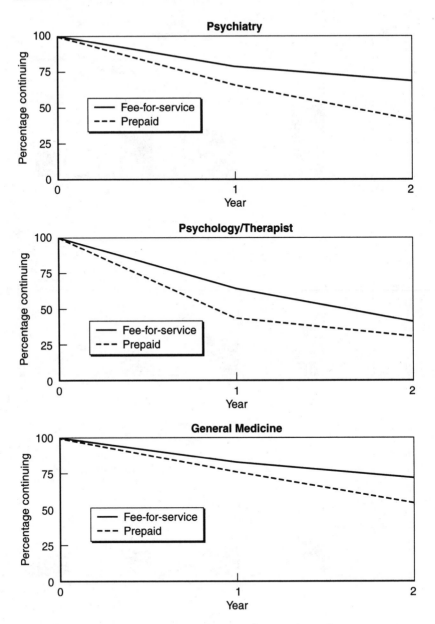

Figure 7.9   Provider Continuity: Percentage Continuing with MOS Clinician

from maintenance therapy). The first case implies a positive correlation between provider switching and patient outcomes and is not necessarily a quality-of-care problem, whereas the second case implies a negative correlation and is definitely a quality-of-care problem. Clearly, both types of cases were present, but the data were not sufficient to distinguish them. A descriptive comparison based on data available from the first follow-up indicated that the reasons for ending a provider relationship in PP were less "voluntary" from the patient's perspective: the provider was no longer available, the patient was referred, or there was a change in the insurance plan. In contrast, FFS patients reported a "voluntary" reason more often: they no longer needed or wanted care.

Chapter Eight

Health Outcomes

Although the analyses of processes of care suggest possible quality-of-care problems, the ultimate test is health outcomes. Maybe patients are treated well enough, considering that many depressed patients improve even without treatment. Relatively little is known about types of depression other than major depression. We therefore first describe clinical outcomes for different types of depression that differ in expected course of illness (for example, major depression, dysthymia, and subthreshold depression) and then analyze whether observed differences in processes of care are accompanied by corresponding differences in health outcomes.

Clinical Outcomes in Actual Practice Settings

The primary focus in the depression research literature is clinical outcomes (for example, remission and recurrence of major depression, symptom counts), as opposed to the functioning outcomes discussed in Chapter 6.[1] Most prior studies of clinical outcomes have focused on patients with major depression, but the MOS also included other types of depression. One important question in the MOS was how dysthymia and subthreshold depressive symptoms compare with major depression.[2]

Figure 8.1 shows the pattern of clinical symptoms and depression spells in follow-up intervals for patients with different types of depression. Patients improved over time and had fewer symptoms and spells in each subsequent follow-up interval, but the level of symptoms

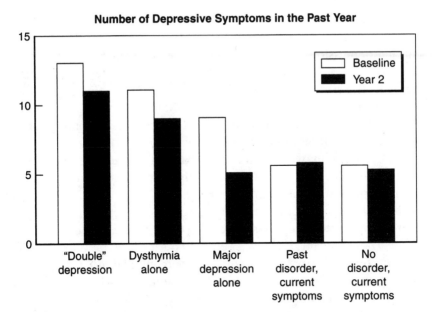

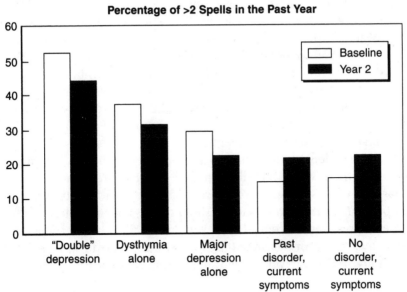

Figure 8.1 Clinical Outcomes for Depressed Patients by Baseline Disorder

remained high even after two years (five to eleven different symptoms in a year, depending on type of depression). Patients with a history of chronic depression (dysthymia), with or without major depression, were particularly likely to have poor clinical outcomes in terms of residual depressive symptoms after two years. Thus, from a clinical outcomes perspective, dysthymia is not a minor form of depression. Patients who initially had subthreshold depressive symptoms (and either a past disorder or just missing criteria for past disorder) showed little improvement over the two years, paralleling the pattern of morbidity outcomes and arguing against the hypothesis that this syndrome represents a transient depression.

Data on major depression also support the conclusion of a high degree of persistent depression. Among those with major depression alone, 41–45 percent of patients remitted during the first year, and 59 percent remitted over two years (41 percent had no remission). Among those with severe double depression, only 41 percent ever remitted from the major depression over two years.

Although depressed patients improved somewhat on average, there was a high level of residual depression and new episodes of depression. Patients with high severity of depressive symptoms also had higher levels of depressive symptoms at two-year follow-up. This is also true for patients with poor functioning and well-being at baseline; in fact, severity of symptoms and level of morbidity explained more variation in clinical outcomes than did type of depressive disorder at baseline, emphasizing the prognostic value of initial morbidity information on depressed patients.

Among patients with dysthymia alone or subthreshold symptoms at baseline, there was a high incidence of major depression over two-year follow-up—more than 50 percent for those with dysthymia and 25 percent for those with subthreshold depression and (almost) lifetime depressive disorder. Thus even the subthreshold groups had outcomes of concern because they were still depressed two years later and were likely to develop major depressive disorder.

Payment Differences in Outcomes

Despite all the public attention that innovations in health care delivery and payment systems receive, little information is available on whether and how they affect health outcomes. The MOS examined differences by payment in outcomes for depressed patients, which provides a better-defined clinical subgroup for outcomes comparison and improves the power to detect such differences.

Figure 8.2 compares FFS and PP in terms of functioning at baseline and year two, where we define payment system by baseline status.[3] The outcome variable is the count of four serious functioning limitations (not able to work, not able to do housework, not able to do strenuous exercise such as lawn mowing, not able to do moderate exercise such as climbing stairs). There was no significant difference in clinical or functioning outcomes by payment type among patients of general medical providers or nonphysician therapists. Clinical symptoms tended to improve regardless of payment or specialty, and

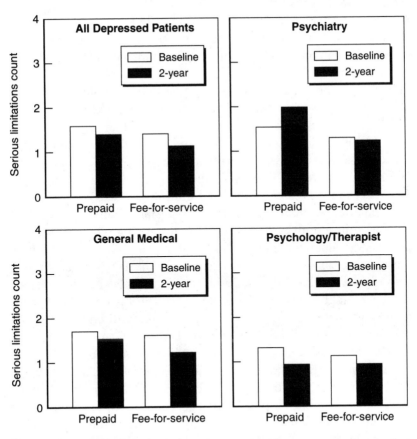

Figure 8.2 Functioning Outcomes by Specialty and Payment

functioning limitations improved little over time for patients of general medical clinicians. This may not be surprising, given that treatment rates were low in that sector regardless of payment. For patients of psychologists and master's-level therapists, counseling rates were similarly high and use of effective antidepressant medication similarly low in both payment systems; in parallel with these process results, there were no significant outcome differences.

In psychiatry, there were highly significant outcome differences in serious functioning limitations between patients initially in PP and patients initially in FFS. PP patients gained new limitations over two years, whereas FFS patients on average improved. The PP patients' gain in limitations is a large effect, comparable to half the patients in the group acquiring a new limitation, such as not being able to work around the house or at a paying job. The level of statistical significance remains high even after adjusting for multiple statistical comparisons. This is therefore not an accidental finding as a consequence of "data mining" (performing comparisons until a significant relationship is found). Nor is it a consequence of a restrictive or misspecified model: the same qualitative findings hold whether we analyzed changes over time in functioning or absolute outcomes at two years; the results are also not affected by other adjustments for sociodemographic factors; and there were no differences in multiple aspects of sickness between payment systems.

These outcome differences should be considered in light of the differences in processes of care and utilization discussed in the previous chapter. Although there were no substantial differences in outpatient utilization by payment system among general medical patients or among nonphysician mental health specialty patients, most savings in terms of visits occurred in the PP psychiatry sector compared with FFS. PP patients of psychiatrists also had significantly shorter patient-provider relationships than FFS patients of psychiatrists, and these relationships were more likely to end for reasons over which the patient had no control. The end of a patient-provider relationship was strongly correlated with discontinuing an antidepressant medication therapy, and PP patients of psychiatrists experienced a much faster decline in medication rates over time than did similar FFS patients, despite starting at similar levels at baseline. The latter finding is likely to be especially important clinically because most patients of psychiatrists had recurrent depression, for which long-term use of antidepressant medication (maintenance therapy) is indicated.

Disruptions in care could also be related to payment plan switching. Among patients of psychiatrists, 28 percent of PP and 9 percent of FFS patients switched payment type by the end of the second follow-up year. Switching was associated with an immediate reduction in utilization, suggesting that patients had difficulty reconnecting with a provider. The difference in functioning outcome for PP and FFS switchers was very large and statistically significant, despite the small sample size. Those switching out of PP care acquired one new limitation over two years on average, whereas those leaving FFS care improved markedly and had one less limitation. It was difficult to determine when exactly a patient deteriorated, but the data suggested that most deteriorations occurred around the time of the switch or maybe slightly earlier.[4]

An important policy question is not only how payment systems compare within each specialty sector, but how they compare for depressed patients overall, across sectors; this is especially important when comparing payment systems that differ in their specialty mix. Averaged across specialty sectors, payment had no significant effects on patient outcomes, as shown in Figure 8.2. This may, however, partly reflect lower statistical precision for the combined sample analysis, despite larger sample size, because of greater variability in outcomes when combining the different specialty groups.[5]

This outcomes analysis also examined differences in outcomes between two different types of PP care, staff-model HMOs and IPAs. IPAs are the fastest growing segment of PP care, and some traditional HMOs are even converting to IPAs, yet there are almost no outcomes studies of IPAs. IPAs are different from HMOs in that plans have no direct control over the practice environment in IPAs, and it is more difficult to monitor and control adherence to practice standards, especially in networks of individual clinicians. Physicians in staff-model HMOs are also more likely to be salaried, whereas a solo practitioner in an IPA may be at full financial risk, which significantly changes incentives.

The sample sizes in the MOS were too small to allow a detailed analysis. Among patients of psychiatrists, each form of PP care had worse functioning than FFS, but the poorest functioning outcomes were in the IPAs. The precision was low, the HMO versus FFS comparison was only significant at .10, and the HMO versus IPA comparison was not significant. We found no differences in general medicine or nonpsychiatry mental health specialty.[6] Nevertheless, these findings, together with geographic differences, indicate that PP health care systems are heterogeneous, suggesting caution in generalizing results from studies of specific practices. Broad labels of PP or FFS are insufficient for capturing meaningful differences in quality of care and outcomes, and the details of clinician incentives (salaried, large risk pools, individual risks), quality monitoring, and practice organization are also important to performance.

Chapter Nine

Cost-Effective Care

As we have seen in the last two chapters, quality of care and patient health outcomes leave much to be desired in typical practices.[1] This has not gone unnoticed; indeed, higher quality of care for depression has become a major clinical care goal nationally. But quality improvement could mean higher total costs, making quality improvement much less attractive in the current policy environment. In fact, the most common observed strategies in today's health care market, such as shifting mental health care from specialty providers to generalists, are driven by cost-containment, not by quality improvement.

An often overlooked criterion that provides a meaningful way to look at the trade-off between quality and costs is *value* of care in terms of health improvements per dollar spent on care. For a health plan or employer, the value of care, or *cost-effectiveness,* should be as important as absolute costs: there is little point in spending money on something that provides no benefits just because it is cheap.

In this chapter, we integrate the utilization, quality-of-care, and health outcomes results to simulate the consequences of different depression treatment patterns for total costs, health outcome, and value of care. This provides new insights into how investing an additional dollar in better quality care can provide the greatest health benefits and how combinations of cost-containment and quality-improvement strategies can be used simultaneously to improve health outcomes while containing costs.

The MOS was not designed for such economic evaluation purposes, making these results more tentative. For example, we have to impute costs from relatively crude treatment data, ignore start-up intervention costs, and use the variation in practice patterns to simulate consequences of improved appropriateness of care. Despite these limitations, the MOS is the best data set that exists today for this purpose because it contains all the necessary information for the analysis in a single, clinically detailed study. In contrast, almost all cost-effectiveness analyses in other areas of health have to rely on literature reviews or expert guesses to obtain the key information on probabilities of treatment, outcomes, structure-process, or process-outcome relationships.

Methods

We use the measurement framework discussed in Chapter 4 as the basis for a structural and analytic model and estimate the empirical relationships among its components (delivery system characteristics, processes of care, and patient outcomes). Through an *indirect analysis* of system-outcome differences (that is, a two-step model showing how delivery system characteristics affect processes and how processes affect outcomes), we also shed light on why different delivery system characteristics lead to different outcomes.

By clarifying the relationships among systems of care, patient casemix, process of care, utilization, and outcomes, this analysis identifies which relationships should be of primary concern to researchers, clinicians, and policymakers. Such an integrated model also has better statistical power to detect clinically important differences in outcomes than a direct "reduced-form" model, which directly compares outcomes by delivery system (as in Chapter 8), because the indirect analysis uses more information on who gets what treatment than the direct analysis.[2]

The advantages of an indirect structural analysis must be balanced against its disadvantages: each model can only be as good as the data and its fit to the substantive questions. For example, we model only the acute phase of depression care in this chapter, not the continuation and maintenance phases.[3] This is an important limitation, considering that Chapters 7 and 8 suggested that important quality-of-care problems exist in the continuation or maintenance phase. The most serious concern, however, the problem of selection biases, is the same in indirect structural and direct "black box" comparisons in an observational study.

We use tools from decision analysis—influence diagrams and decision trees—to build the structural model. The parameters of the model (the relationships among the components of our measurement framework) are estimated statistically from MOS. This statistical analysis also helps to determine the final structure of the model by allowing us to prune relationships that seem to be of secondary importance. We first estimate the relationship among delivery structures (payment, specialty) and processes of care (antidepressant medication, counseling, and minor tranquilizer use) and then the linkage of these processes to outcomes (changes in functioning limitations and imputed costs). We calculated annual treatment costs based on outpatient mental health care utilization and psychotropic medication because there was no significant association between other types of utilization and the processes of care analyzed.[4] This also suggests that cost-offsets in general medical costs through more appropriate care for depression are unlikely to be a major factor.

The model is shown in the influence diagram of Figure 9.1. The arrows between the nodes represent significant relationships (conditioning) in which the state of the conditioned event (pointed to by the

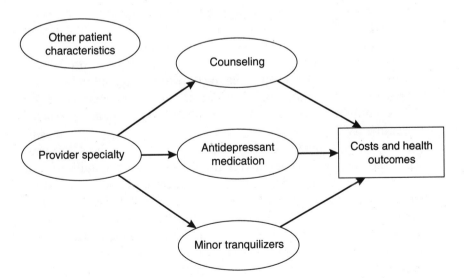

Figure 9.1 Model of Care for Depression

arrow) depends on the state of the conditioning event (the origin of the arrow). The probability of prescribing medication, for example, depends on provider specialty. The absence of arrows between components means that there was no statistically significant direct relationship. For example, after controlling for patient characteristics and provider specialty, we found that counseling did not predict the use of antidepressant medication and vice versa. For graphical clarity, we excluded the arrows emanating from patient characteristics (initial physical and psychological health status, ethnicity, gender, marital status, age, education), but we controlled for those factors when necessary. We can only give details on some of our results, and the parameters and findings discussed here have a limited scope: acute care under PP care for the most severely depressed patients.[5]

The three outcome dimensions are:

- Health: change in number of serious functioning limitations;[6]
- Costs: imputed treatment costs for depression; and
- Value of care: costs for reducing one functioning limitation.

Processes of Care and Outcomes: The Model Parameters

The probability that a severely depressed patient in a PP plan visits a general medical clinician, a psychiatrist, or another mental health specialist as a regular source of care is given in the first row of Table 9.1.[7] The next three rows give the parameters for the key process-of-care measures. The final row gives the detection rate, but detection is not part of our simulation model because it has no independent *direct* effect on outcome. Detection has only an *indirect* effect as a predictor of treatments.[8]

Table 9.2 presents the estimated process-outcomes links. We estimate outcomes associated with regular use of minor tranquilizers, not with avoidance of such use, which is the indicator of appropriate care, because minor tranquilizers are not of established efficacy in depression (Depression Guidelines Panel, 1993b). The effectiveness of treatments does not differ significantly by specialty, but the probability of treatment does. For example, the effect of antidepressant medication or counseling does not differ by specialty. Specialty differences in outcomes are due primarily to different rates of effective treatment.

Table 9.1   Probability of Type of Treatment for Severely Depressed Patients

Probability of process of care	Psychiatry	General medicine	Other mental health specialty
Probability that treating provider is	.31	.44	.25
Probability that patient uses appropriate antidepressant medication[a]	.44	.21	.16
Probability that patient uses minor tranquilizer regularly[a]	.57	.36	.34
Probability that patient receives counseling for depression at baseline[b]	.87	.37	.84
Probability that patient is detected as being depressed[b, c]	.90	.49	.91

Source: Sturm and Wells (1995).
a. Psychiatry is statistically significant from other two groups ($p < 0.05$).
b. General medical is statistically significant from other two groups ($p < 0.05$).
c. Detection is not directly associated with health outcomes or costs and not part of the simulation model.

This is an assumption of the model that is empirically based on data from the MOS, but that some critics may question.

For the sickest patients, appropriate care for depression is significantly correlated with better outcomes in the context of care as usual. Counseling for depression and use of appropriate antidepressant medication are jointly significant at $p = 0.01$ and substantially very important: compared with no treatment, counseling and antidepressant medication provided together lead to ninety-five fewer serious limitations in one hundred patients, supporting the validity of the processes measures as indicators of quality of care. Confidence intervals are fairly wide, however, and, more important, the quantitative relationships changed when we changed the model for sensitivity analyses, although the qualitative finding that appropriate care improves outcomes was robust. To reflect this sensitivity, we report a

Table 9.2   Functioning and Cost Outcomes Associated with Processes of Care for Severely Depressed Patients

Process of care	Number of functioning limitations reduced	Direct mental health treatment costs ($)		
		P	GM	OMH
Counseling and appropriate antidepressant medication use	+0.68	4,200	1,755	2,940
Counseling, appropriate use of antidepressant medication, and regular minor tranquilizer use	+0.48	4,425	1,980	3,165
Counseling only	+0.40	3,505	1,310	2,500
Counseling and regular minor tranquilizer use	+0.20	3,730	1,535	2,725
Appropriate antidepressant medication use only	+0.01	2,660	1,070	1,980
Appropriate antidepressant medication use and regular minor tranquilizer use	−0.19	2,885	1,295	2,205
No depression treatment	−0.27	2,125	630	1,360
Regular minor tranquilizer use only	−0.47	2,250	855	1,585
Joint significance test	$p = 0.03$	$p < 0.01$		

Source: Sturm and Wells (1995).

Note: Reduction in functioning limitations is scaled −4 to +4, with a more positive score indicating more improvement (more limitations removed); direct mental health treatment costs are imputed outpatient costs including visits and medications. P = psychiatry; GM = general medicine; OMH = other mental health specialty.

range for outcomes findings in Tables 9.4 and 9.5, rather than a point estimate. This range covers three different assumptions:

1. that our estimates are correct;
2. that changes in minor tranquilizer use have no effect on functional status; and

3. that the effect of counseling and effective antidepressant medication is identical and equal to the average of our two estimates.

Treatment increases mental health care utilization and costs, regardless of specialty. Counseling for depression at the screening visit is associated with an additional 11 mental health visits in the next year, compared with no counseling. Use of appropriate antidepressant medication is associated on average with 4.5 subsequent mental health visits in a year, plus medication costs. This is roughly consistent with practice guideline recommendations about starting and monitoring use of such medications. Regular use of minor tranquilizers, however, is not significantly associated with increased mental health visits.

Table 9.2 also gives the imputed costs of care associated with treatment, by type of provider at baseline (screening visit). For example, the P column gives the outpatient costs of patients of psychiatrists.

Simulating Quality Improvement and Patient Shifting

To demonstrate the effect of the trend away from specialty care, we simulate the cost and outcome implications of the actual mix in PP care in the study period (shown in the first row of Table 9.1), and a greater shift away from psychiatric care, that is, probabilities of .15, .60, and .25 for being in psychiatric, general medical, or other mental health therapist practice.

Our heuristic for markedly improving quality of care is to reduce inappropriate care by about two-thirds. This leads to the increases in treatment rates for each provider sector in Table 9.3. We consider three nested quality improvement strategies that reflect a clinical rationale for changing practice: first focus on treatments with demonstrated efficacy that are simple and inexpensive (antidepressant medication in this application), then on treatments with demonstrated efficacy that are more difficult to provide and require more substantial changes in practice style (counseling), and finally on debatable issues (reducing minor tranquilizer use).

A cost-effectiveness analyst would present results somewhat differently (two very good recent introductions to those methods in health care are Eisenberg, 1989, and Kamlet, 1992). First, the analyst would focus on the most cost-effective intervention, which is reducing the use of an expensive but ineffective therapy. In our case, this is regular

Table 9.3   Definitions and Target Goals for Three Levels of Improved Appropriateness of Care, by Specialty

Definition	Target goal[a] (percentage of severely depressed patients visiting the practice who meet process criteria)		
	Psychiatry	General medicine	Other mental health specialty
Level 1: Use antidepressant medication in a therapeutic daily dosage and 4–5 follow-up visits	70	70	70
Level 2: Level 1 goals achieved plus provide counseling for depression and 11–12 additional "mental health" visits	95	70	95
Level 3: Level 2 goals achieved plus limit regular use of minor tranquilizers[b]	10	10	10

Source: Sturm and Wells (1995).
a. The target goal refers to the new process introduced at that level only.
b. No more than 10 percent of patients will use minor tranquilizers regularly.

minor tranquilizer use. Second, the analyst would target the process of care with the next lowest cost-effectiveness ratio (CE; the additional expenditures necessary to remove one additional functioning limitation). This could be either counseling or antidepressant medication (our results are not conclusive), yet most practices would first consider increases in antidepressant medication.

Why do we deviate from the standard way of presenting cost-effectiveness results? Cost-effectiveness analysis is a tool that provides new insights, not a formula that provides a final answer. Many aspects of a decision problem require judgment and reflect dimensions that are not modeled formally. Adapting the presentation of results to reflect these issues can improve the relevance of such analyses to practitioners. For example, there appear to be disagreements among clinicians about minor tranquilizers, making it unlikely that reducing their use would become a first universally accepted goal, and we therefore considered it as the last element of a comprehensive strategy. There are also short-term costs involved in moving toward these new practice patterns, but our numbers only simulate the implications of practice patterns that have already changed. While our numbers represent the relevant long-term perspective, these short-term interventions costs are likely to be higher for changing counseling patterns in general medicine than for improving antidepressant medication management.

Costs, Health Outcomes, and Value of Care

The first row in each section (a-c) of Table 9.4 shows the performance, in terms of costs and functioning outcomes, of current patterns of treatment for severely depressed patients in PP care for each specialty sector considered individually. The next three rows provide total treatment costs per patient, the average in functioning limitations (on a −4 to +4 scale, with a more positive score indicating more limitations removed), and the cost-effectiveness ratio for the three nested quality-improvement strategies. The cost-effectiveness ratio is the marginal costs of removing one additional functioning limitation, over care as usual. A comparison of the first rows of Tables 9.4a–c shows that under current practice patterns, the lowest costs, but also the worst outcomes, are in the general medical sector; the highest costs, but also the best outcomes, occur in psychiatry.

In the general medical sector (Table 9.4a), under care as usual, there is a slight deterioration in functioning, although this is substantially better than the deterioration expected in the absence of any treatment. Each level of quality improvement has the potential of substantially improving patient outcomes. The estimated health improvement under Level 1 compared with care as usual is similar to removing an additional fourteen to twenty-four serious functioning limitations from one hundred severely depressed patients. The improvement is even more dramatic, affecting all three types of processes of care (Level 3). The cost-effectiveness ratios for improving processes of care are in the $1,000 range, meaning that the marginal cost of removing one additional functional limitation through higher appropriate treatment rates is around $1,000.

In psychiatry (which already has more appropriate treatment, better outcomes, and higher treatment costs), the degree of additional

Table 9.4   Simulation of Quality Improvement[a]

Table 9.4a General medicine	Costs per patient ($)	Improvement in functioning	Cost-effectiveness ratio[b]
General medical care as usual	1,060	−.04	—
Level 1: Increase use of appropriate antidepressant medication	1,270	.10–.20	870–1,500
Level 2: Increase both antidepressants and counseling	1,490	.32–.35	1,100–1,200
Level 3: Increase antidepressants and counseling, reduce minor tranquilizers	1,430	.32–.43	790–1030

Table 9.4b Psychiatry	Costs per patient ($)	Improvement in functioning	Cost-effectiveness ratio[c]
Psychiatric care as usual	3,760	.32	—
Level 1: Increase use of appropriate antidepressant medication	3,940	.40–.44	1,500–2,250
Level 2: Increase both antidepressants and counseling	4,050	.45–.48	1,810–2,230
Level 3: Increase antidepressants and counseling, reduce minor tranquilizers	3,940	.45–.67	510–1,380

Table 9.4   (continued)

Table 9.4c Other mental health specialty	Costs per patient ($)	Improvement in functioning	Cost-effectiveness ratio[d]
Other mental health care as usual	2,500	.27	—
Level 1: Increase use of appropriate antidepressant medication	2,840	.42–.52	1,360–2,270
Level 2: Increase both antidepressants and counseling	2,960	.49–.58	1,480–2,090
Level 3: Increase antidepressants and counseling, reduce minor tranquilizers	2,910	.49–.67	1,030–1,860

Source: Sturm and Wells (1995).

a. Range of outcome changes and cost-effectiveness ratios corresponds to the three qualitatively different assumptions about process-outcome associations.

b. Calculated relative to current care in the general medical sector; the ratio gives the additional cost to remove one additional functional limitation; −.04 is 4 new limitations among 100 patients.

c. Calculated relative to current care in psychiatry; the low cost-effectiveness ratio of the combined QI strategy is due to substantial cost-savings through avoidance of minor tranquilizers.

d. Calculated relative to current care in other mental health specialty.

outcome improvement (over care as usual) that can be achieved at each level of process change is more moderate, and the cost-effectiveness ratios for Levels 1 and 2 process changes are close to $2,000—twice the cost-effectiveness ratio for these levels of process changes in general medicine (Table 9.4b). At Level 3, however, the cost-effectiveness ratio is comparable to that for general medicine, owing to reduction of minor tranquilizer use, which is prevalent under usual care in psychiatry. The increase in total costs per patient at Level 3 over care as usual is under $200 in psychiatry, that is, less than a 10 percent increase in costs. The comparable amount for general medicine is $400 because of the greater change in counseling we simulated.

For patients of psychologists and master's-level therapists, most of what can be achieved in improved outcomes and cost-effectiveness is achieved at Level 1 (Table 9.4c), because these patients are already counseled and few receive minor tranquilizers. The cost-effectiveness ratios are in the range of $1,000–$2,000 (similar to psychiatry).

Practices and plans may set quality-improvement goals for the practice as a whole, rather than for one specialty sector. Accordingly, we evaluated the impact of quality improvement and shifting specialty mix across specialty sectors (Table 9.5). We present the cost-effectiveness ratio relative to no care (the average costs of improving one functioning limitation), because the cost-effectiveness ratios compared with care as usual have different interpretations depending on whether costs under improved care are greater or lower than the status quo. We assumed that "no care" was equivalent to zero treatment costs and the same outcome (a decrement equal to 0.27 new functioning limitations) as for patients in care who receive no treatment for depression.

The right-hand side of Table 9.5 shows the effects of quality improvement for the system as a whole under current specialty mix. The current system spends more than $5,000 to remove one functioning limitation (first row of Table 9.5). This is 2.5 to 5 times the marginal costs ($1,000–$2,000) of removing an additional functioning limitation under quality improvement. Thus quality improvement improves the value of care, because the lower marginal costs of additional health improvements drive down the average costs of health improvement. All levels of quality improvement raise total costs of care by 10–20 percent.

The right-hand side of Table 9.5 presents the parallel results under a shift toward general medical care, that is, the trend in the health care market. Without quality improvement, the shift toward general medicine reduces costs, worsens functioning, and leaves average cost largely unaffected (compare the left-hand and right-hand sides of the first row). Under shifted specialty mix, each level of quality improvement still raises costs and improves health outcomes; but the specialty mix shift offsets the increase in costs due to quality improvement, and the quality improvement offsets the decline in outcomes due to specialty mix shift. Specifically, costs for most levels on the right-hand side of Table 9.5 are lower than the current treatment costs of $2,250. Consequently, it is possible that combining quality improvement with

Table 9.5 Effects for the System (across Specialty Sectors) of Improved Appropriateness and of a Specialty Shift to General Medical Care for Severely Depressed Patients

Process of care	Specialty mix as in MOS			New specialty mix		
	Costs per patient ($)	Functioning limitations reduced	CE[a]	Costs per patient ($)	Functioning limitations reduced	CE[a]
Care as usual	2,250	.15	5,360	1,825	.09	5,070
Level 1: Increase use of appropriate antidepressant medication	2,490	.27–.35	4,020–4,610	2,060	.23–.32	3,490–4,120
Level 2: Increase both antidepressants and counseling	2,650	.40–.45	3,680–3,950	2,240	.38–.43	3,200–3,450
Level 3: Increase antidepressants and counseling, reduce minor tranquilizers	2,580	.40–.56	3,110–3,850	2,180	.38–.53	2,730–3,350
Level 3a: Increase antidepressants and counseling, reduce minor tranquilizers only in general medical	2,420	.31–.36	3,840–4,170	2,050	.31–.37	3,200–3,530

Source: Sturm and Wells (1995).
Note: Specialty mix in MOS for severely depressed patients (sickest quartile according to overall psychological health): 44 percent general medicine, .31 percent psychiatry, 25 percent other mental health specialties. Simulated "new" mix: 60 percent general medicine, 15 percent psychiatry, 25 percent other mental health specialties.
a. Average cost of removing one functioning limitation (cost-effectiveness ratio relative to no care, assuming $0 costs and −.27 deterioration).

the trend away from specialty care could contain treatment costs but improve health outcomes, increasing the value of care. The same qualitative conclusions hold even if quality improvement is limited to general medical practices (Level 3a), but at lower levels of improvements in outcomes and value of care. These results assume that relative specialty costs and treatment effectiveness remain stable, that is, at current levels.

What We Can Learn from This Analysis

More appropriate care for depression, roughly reflecting key recommendations of clinical practice guidelines, is likely to improve functioning outcomes and to increase greatly the value of health care spending in terms of health benefits. The costs of removing an additional functioning limitation are substantially smaller than the average costs that plans currently incur to remove one, making quality improvement a high-value strategy despite increases in utilization (and costs) associated with better quality of care. In contrast, shifting patients to general medical providers under current treatment patterns in each sector lowers costs of care but also leads to poorer functioning outcomes and has little effect on the value of care.

Combining these two approaches, quality improvement and shifting, can achieve all goals simultaneously: reduce total costs, improve health outcomes, and increase the value of care. This is a very fortunate situation, but it reflects a more general principle: if there are several competing goals, one needs a mix of several different policy levers or strategies to address all of them. There rarely is a dominating strategy that achieves every goal. Cost-containment strategies are unlikely to improve the quality of care, and quality improvement strategies are similarly unlikely to contain costs.

Through our simulation model, we can trace out the trade-off between costs and quality. What are the minimum levels of quality improvements in general medicine to counter the adverse effects of the common cost-containment strategy of shifting to general medicine? A plan that shifts an additional 5 percent of its severely depressed patients from psychiatric to general medical care needs to increase the percentage of patients using appropriate antidepressant medication in general medical practice by about 18 percentage points (from 21 percent to almost 40 percent) to maintain the same outcomes as plans that do not change their specialty mix. Shifting 10 percent of the patients requires increasing appropriate medication rates to about 50 percent in general medical practices. Larger shifts (>15 percent) or attempts to improve outcomes substantially over current care as usual require more comprehensive strategies, such as Levels 2 and 3.

Where should a PP plan spend its next dollar for higher quality care? The most cost-effective improvements are available in the general medical sector, although quality improvement strategies that include reducing regular minor tranquilizer use in psychiatry could also be very cost-effective. Regular use of minor tranquilizers has a negative effect on the cost-effectiveness of psychiatric care because of their cost and their negative or neutral associations with functioning outcome: in order to be as cost-effective as general medical care as usual, the psychiatrist rate per visit would have to drop to about $80, which probably even the most cost-conscious PP plan cannot achieve, except possibly through relying on group therapy. If one first focused on reducing minor tranquilizer use in psychiatry to 10 percent, however, then psychiatry provides better value of care than general medicine as usual for $100 a visit. In other words, excess regular minor tranquilizer use in PP psychiatric practices has the same adverse effect on value of care as increasing the cost for each visit by $20.

Our focus on direct depression treatment costs could be criticized as too narrow a cost perspective, but we did not find any effect of depression treatments on the use of nonmental health care visits or on inpatient utilization (either for mental health or for medical reasons). If a cost-offset effect exists (Mumford et al., 1984), it was too small for us to detect, and any such effect would be overwhelmed by the increased costs of more appropriate care. We point out, however, that measurement error can result in positive cost-offset effects in data sets that cannot distinguish between mental health and physical health reasons for a general medical visit: patients receiving mental health care in the general medical sector may show up as higher users of medical care in such studies than patients receiving care from mental health specialists, but it is really their "mental health" general medical visits that are increased. In our analyses, such visits were included as mental health visits.

Improved care for depression is likely to reduce indirect costs of depression, although there is no research in this area as yet that would permit us to assess the overall impact. Mintz et al. (1992) found that work outcomes in terms of unemployment and on-the-job performance improved when treatment for depression was symptomatically effective, although they did not obtain a monetary estimate of this effect. We explored this issue using MOS data on family income over time. The reduction of one functional limitation is associated with an increase of annual earned family income of around $2,000 for the sickest depressed patients. Thus even if the patient's family were to pay the full marginal cost ($1,000–$2,000) of removing an additional limitation under improved quality of care, it would be a net monetary gain for them—in addition to all the advantages of better health. From a public finance perspective, the increase in employment and earnings associated with better care is likely to increase tax revenue and lower unemployment and welfare payments. This broader perspective suggests that quality of care for depression may currently be at a socially inefficient level.

Chapter Ten

Depression in a Changing Health Care Environment

The U.S. health care system is quickly changing, but are we moving in the right direction? What do different payment strategies, quality-improvement interventions, or an increased reliance on primary care gatekeepers mean in terms of outcomes or costs for mental health problems?

Studying Effectiveness

For policy purposes, we need to know whether care affects outcomes in typical practices (its effectiveness), and this is best determined in an observational study using specific tracer conditions. This approach is very different from clinical studies that demonstrate whether a specific treatment can affect outcomes in a controlled setting (efficacy). Our policy focus requires a compromise in the clinical precision of data compared with clinical trials. But at the same time the tracer condition approach goes beyond typical policy studies in that it allows us to study many clinical details, such as the appropriateness of medications.

The effectiveness of care in actual practice settings is likely to differ from the demonstrated efficacy in clinical trials, and we cannot rely on process measures to compare quality of care with the expectation that this implies known outcome differences. Instead, we must complement data on processes of care with primary data collection on health outcomes. We consider health outcomes an important complement because relying on them alone is not without problems either.

Health outcomes are difficult to measure and not sensitive enough to detect substantial differences at standard significance levels with commonly available sample sizes. Comparisons with low statistical power could easily be abused to "prove" the absence of a significant difference and justify promotion of a cheaper, but possibly less effective, alternative.

Despite being quite complex, this health-oriented perspective still lacks one major social outcome: health care costs. So long as one focuses on health outcomes in isolation, quality of care can never be high enough. But quality improvement generally means higher total costs, and many strategies in today's health care market, such as shifting mental health care from specialty providers to generalists, reflect a focus on costs and ignore health outcomes—which is easy to do, as some costs data are usually available whereas outcomes data are not. Our study of value of care or cost-effectiveness combines both economic and health perspectives. Our results are preliminary— the MOS unfortunately paid less attention to measuring economic concepts—but this intersection of economic and health services research will become much more common in the future.

Finally, health care is inefficient when sick individuals do not receive appropriate care for their health problem or when others receive treatment they do not need. A tracer approach mainly limits us to analyzing the first type of error because it identifies individuals with a specific health problem. Overuse, the second type of error, is generally believed to be less of a quality-of-care problem, but it certainly has cost implications. Unfortunately, screening patients for not having specific health problems that could benefit from treatments they receive is quite problematic. For example, we cannot be confident that treating minor depression as if it were major depression is inappropriate. Consequently, almost all research fails to balance the two types of errors and is biased in favor of health care that reduces undertreatment, regardless of the magnitude of the second type of error. The MOS is no exception in this regard, although we can at least study use of medications that are not first-line treatments for depression.

The need for effectiveness data in administrative and clinical decision-making also has design implications for clinical trials. First, the generalizability of traditional clinical trials that sample from the specialty sector and exclude patients on the basis of comorbidities is questionable; the MOS showed that the typical depressed patient has multiple comorbidities and receives care in the general medical sector. Second, we found that depression is a chronic illness in terms of morbidity, and this chronicity is not limited to persons with dysthymic disorder, but includes a high percentage of persons with so-called time-limited depressions (major depressive disorder and subthreshold depressive symptoms). Unfortunately, clinical trials rarely follow patients for more than a few months, although recent studies suggest that health benefits of treatments for depression may only be short-term (Katon et al., 1995). Further research is needed on how treatment and management strategies can minimize long-term disability. Such studies should evaluate costs as well as long-term morbidity outcomes. Given the high percentage of practice patients with recurrent depression, research on the long-run effectiveness of general medical counseling for depression, as well as brief forms of psychotherapy in the mental health specialty sector, is especially needed.

Impacts of Different Types of Depression

We showed that depression (major depression, dysthymia, and subthreshold symptoms) is an important public health problem because it is often poorly treated even though it is prevalent among outpatients and affects individual functioning and well-being at least as much as common chronic medical conditions. These three forms of depression are generally perceived to be very different: major depression is considered a serious problem, whereas dysthymic disorder and subthreshold systems are considered to be of minor importance. We found these assumptions to be incorrect, because dysthymic disorder is more disabling than major depression, even though it is less common. Unfortunately, treatments for dysthymic disorder have been much less studied, so there are limited data on which to base resource allocation decisions for this condition. Our results cast doubt on the wisdom of singling out major depression as the only unipolar disorder to achieve coverage.

Subthreshold symptoms are often characterized as transient and having little impact, but we found that they are much more prevalent than depressive disorders, although they have lower levels of associated morbidity. Treatment implications for subthreshold depression are uncertain, and we found no evidence for effectiveness of antidepressant medication or counseling in less severe depressions. This could mean that subthreshold symptoms should be a low priority for health care resource allocation, but this need not be the case, as even small effects of treatment on morbidity can be of social importance for highly prevalent conditions that strongly affect indirect costs. In making this allocation decision, one would need to understand the total social cost implications of treating subthreshold depression, but the costs of such a study may be prohibitive, given the large sample sizes needed as a result of the heterogeneity of subthreshold depression and the relatively small treatment effects.

Differences in Payment Systems and Provider Specialty Sectors

Despite all the attention paid to biased selection, we found little evidence that depressed patients differ between payment systems in any aspect of their depression severity, health status, or functioning. The absence of health-related biased selection does not mean that patients are identical, of course. Patients with a preference for intensive care—regardless of their clinical status—are likely to select themselves into plans that permit easy access to specialty care, typically FFS plans, and patients with a preference for more limited care and lower costs are likely to prefer PP managed care. Such selections affect our interpretation of the extent to which patient preferences versus system characteristics shape utilization. Financing systems could also differ in their enrollee pool—we did not study nonusers of services—which could give a plan with healthier enrollees an advantage because costs per enrollee would be lower.

Provider specialty is a different dimension of policy interest, and here we need to pay special attention to health-related selection effects because probability and type of treatment depend on sickness and because psychiatrists treat the sickest patients in terms of psychological health. Obviously, we cannot just compare the average patient across sectors; rather, we need to select comparable groups or achieve comparability through statistical controls. This is always a problem for observational studies, but the MOS included a comprehensive health inventory for such adjustments.

To compare quality of care, we contrasted payment and specialty groups in three clinical processes: detection, counseling, and psychotropic medication. We also analyzed utilization and continuity of care. The differences in process of care by specialty sector were always great and robust to different ways to control for sickness differences. Thus we believe that our specialty conclusions are reliable even in the absence of an experimental assignment of patients.

Detection

The widespread concern about under-recognition of mental health conditions in the general medical sector requires some qualifications. First, it is effective treatment that improves depression, not detection alone. Being detected does not guarantee that a patient will receive appropriate treatment: many detected depressed patients in the MOS received medications that were at best of questionable value for their depression. It is quite possible to have both high detection rates and poor quality of care if organizational and financial incentives reduce the use of appropriate clinical treatments. In such cases, increased detection rates channel more patients into an ineffective course of clinical treatment and may be one reason for the disappointing health outcome results of interventions focusing solely on detection.

The second qualification concerns the clinician time trade-off between screening for different types of disease conditions. It is not clear that emphasizing one particular condition makes patients better off if it comes at the expense of poorer quality of care for other conditions. Unfortunately, the opportunity costs of improving detection for one condition have not yet been studied.

Studying detection of a specific treatable condition provides a first cut at understanding quality of care. We clearly see a major difference between mental health specialists, who detect most depressed patients, and general medical providers, who detect only about 50 percent of their depressed patients. Detection rates were slightly lower under PP than FFS general medical care, but the main difference was between general medical and specialty providers.

Psychotropic Medication

We found three general problems with medication management in all practice settings: the rates of antidepressant medication use were low, subtherapeutic dosages among users were common, and minor tranquilizers were used more often than antidepressants. The low rate of antidepressant medication use in general medical practices was not surprising and reflected the low rate of detection. Antidepressant medication use was similarly low among patients of nonphysician mental health specialists, however, and those patients encountered an additional problem in that antidepressant medication was not targeted to psychologically sicker patients, suggesting a lack of coordination between the nonphysician therapist and the prescribing physician. In contrast, psychiatrists were more likely both to prescribe antidepressant medications and to respond to patient sickness: about half their patients with high severity and just under a third of those with low severity used an antidepressant medication. But even in psychiatry the medication rates appear rather low in the light of practice guidelines recommending that severely depressed patients receive antidepressant medications in the absence of contraindications or a failure to respond to adequate trials. In addition, subtherapeutic dosages of antidepressant medications were common in all practices.

More patients received minor tranquilizers than antidepressant medications, and treatment with both types of medications was not uncommon. Minor tranquilizer use was more common in psychiatry than in general medicine even for comparable patient groups, which contradicts the common belief that specialists are better at avoiding inefficient medications. Overall, our results indicate that there is a need to review clinical practice patterns against accepted standards in the field, and that specialists, not just general medical providers, should be the target of efforts to improve medication management.

Another surprising finding was that PP practices had an even higher rate of minor tranquilizer use than FFS practices, which contradicts the often-heard claim that PP care is more efficient because it reduces unnecessary care. Managed-care clinicians have suggested to us that pressures to reduce costs and increase caseloads lead to the use of minor tranquilizers as a substitute for visits. Maybe clinicians unfamiliar with appropriate care for depression are also more susceptible to advertising or patient suggestions for a specific medication and use a minor tranquilizer prescription as a quick way out of an awkward decision problem, which could explain the use of costly brand-name minor tranquilizers.

The extensive marketing and publicity surrounding new antidepressant medications such as Prozac, which were only used in the

MOS follow-up years, may have tilted the balance toward antidepressants in recent years, as well as increasing rates of treatment. But treatment rates appear to have increased relatively little, and the underlying causes of poor quality of care are unlikely to have disappeared, making medication management—increasing the use of appropriate antidepressant medication and reducing regular use of minor tranquilizers—one of the most promising targets of quality-improvement interventions.

Counseling

Psychotherapy is the second commonly used treatment for depression, but it is difficult to measure in actual care settings. We had to rely on provider self-report of whether or not at least very brief counseling occurred, followed by additional visits.

Not surprisingly, almost all (80 percent) depressed patients of mental health specialists received some counseling, primarily individual psychotherapy. In contrast, only a third of the patients in general medical practices (including those with unrecognized depression) received even very brief counseling for depression, and rates of counseling were significantly lower under PP than FFS plans in this sector. Training and practice constraints are undoubtedly a central reason for the lower rates of counseling in general medical practices, but patient preferences also matter, as patients wanting psychotherapy select themselves into specialty care.

Usual counseling style differed primarily by specialty, not by payment, and was more intensive and psychodynamically oriented in the specialty sector and briefer and more advice-oriented in the general medical sector. Specialists provide what is typically called psychotherapy, whereas medical providers deliver a more general form of medical counseling. Most mental health specialists would claim that medical counseling is less effective than formal psychotherapy, although there are virtually no comparative data. Counseling had a significant beneficial effect on patient functioning, suggesting that some form of counseling specifically for depression is helpful. We found no significant differences in the effect of counseling on patient functioning among provider types, indicating that provider type and the particular form of counseling are likely to be of secondary importance compared with whether or not any counseling occurs.

Payment Systems and Health Outcomes

The intensity of mental health care visits was lower in PP than in FFS plans, but there were no major differences in health outcomes on average. PP psychiatry and general medical practices, however, showed some evidence of poorer quality of care for depressed patients than their FFS counterparts in a variety of process and health impact measures (detection, counseling, use of minor tranquilizers, continuation of antidepressant medication, provider continuity, and functioning outcomes). Thus our finding of no average differences in functioning outcomes by payment is not as reassuring as it otherwise might be.

The greatest differences between PP and FFS patients in processes of care and utilization were among patients of psychiatrists, who were also the sickest patients in both payment systems. Among PP psychiatry patients, we observed a more rapid decline in antidepressant medication usage over time, shorter patient-provider relationships, and a higher use of minor tranquilizers—all of which were reflected in significantly worse functioning outcomes under PP care. Thus PP care appears to have problems for the sickest patients who visit psychiatrists, and quality-improvement efforts should not necessarily be limited to the general medical sector.

Discontinuities in patient-provider relationships could either cause or result from a quality problem. The MOS focused on the acute phase of depression, not on maintenance treatment, and we cannot determine the cost, health benefit, or value of maintenance therapy in usual care. This information requires longitudinal studies assessing long-term economic and morbidity outcomes under alternative practice strategies, such as acute-care medical models versus long-term coordinated care models or biological treatments versus psychosocial care.

FFS care did not distinguish itself in terms of quality of care either, despite much higher costs. Further, FFS practice is much more aggressively managed in most parts of the United States now than during the MOS study period, especially in the sites studied in the MOS. If such management within FFS has led to process-of-care results similar to those in PP care in the late 1980s, then quality improvement could be an equally high priority across current PP and FFS plans. Another major change in the managed-care market has been the rapid growth of managed-care companies specializing in mental health and sub-stance abuse services ("carve-out" management). This industry has argued that the special attention to mental health services within a separate company permits both high quality of care and cost reduc-tion, but there have been virtually no rigorous comparative data. Thus the main policy question for depression care currently is not whether we should promote one type of payment or managed-care system, but how to achieve more cost-effective care for depression overall.

Making Care More Cost-Effective

If we want to spend our depression care dollars efficiently, an impor-tant criterion should be amount of improvement in morbidity for each additional health care dollar spent. The current returns on money spent on depression care seem low: each reduction in one functioning limitation costs about $5,000 under care as usual in PP care and even more in FFS. The return is low because many patients consume resources that do not help them with their depression, not because treatment for depression per se is expensive.

Inefficient care exists in all sectors, and no specialty sector provides care of particularly high value. Care for depression is much cheaper in general medical practice than in psychiatry, but health outcomes are worse because general medical patients are less likely to receive appropriate care during their visits, whereas the better outcomes in psychiatry are accompanied by greater use of ineffective minor tran-quilizers and high visit costs. As a consequence, the trend of shifting patients to general medical providers can reduce costs, but it also deteriorates outcomes and does little to improve the value of care.

In contrast to shifting patients, quality-improvement raises the value of care because the marginal cost of removing one additional functional limitation through more appropriate treatment is much lower than what plans are currently paying on average for removing one limitation. Although achieving quality improvement raises the value of care (which we consider to be cost-effective), it also raises total costs of mental health care somewhat. Combining both strate-gies of quality improvement and shifting specialty mix has the poten-tial to contain costs and improve outcomes or even reduce costs and improve outcomes simultaneously, however: specialty shifting reduces total costs, whereas quality improvement raises costs, but less than it improves outcomes and cost-effectiveness.

Although it is theoretically possible to improve outcomes and value of care and contain or lower costs of care, this possibility rests on several assumptions: that quality improvement can be achieved, that costs of improved general medical care for depression will remain substantially lower than costs of specialty care, and that sicker patients can be shifted to general medical practice. Further, the absolute magnitude of the gains that can be achieved in outcomes or value of care through quality improvement depends on how high prevailing treatment rates are prior to quality improvement.

Regarding the first assumption, early studies of quality improvement are not very encouraging, but their focus on detection seems the wrong priority for cost-effective care, which requires improved treatment of identified cases first. Accomplishing substantial improvements in quality of care probably requires changing financial incentives, such as reimbursing medical counseling for depression, and achieving a greater consensus among primary care providers that treating depression is a priority. Poor quality of care for depression may be a "bad habit," and a cultural and environmental change may be necessary to facilitate improved quality of care. New studies are currently focusing on the consequences of improving quality of care for depression in primary care, and new information on what can be achieved with more comprehensive change strategies should be available within the next five years.

Regarding the second assumption, we think it is likely that improved general medical care will remain cheaper than specialty care, even though the difference is likely to shrink. General medical visit duration may go up to accommodate more assessment and treatment of depression, but our analyses already assumed longer than average visits. To remain competitive, mental health specialty practices could lower their price by shifting to less expensive therapists or less expensive forms of therapies, such as group rather than individual therapy or shorter or fewer sessions. These trends are already occurring under managed care, and such competition also improves a plan's performance in the absolute cost dimension.

Regarding the third assumption, we assumed that patients can be shifted to general medicine. In the short run, the extent of shifting is limited by patient and provider preferences, the supply of general medical providers, competing demands for the attention of providers, and limited practice resources to accommodate depressed patients. Patients might prefer specialty care, and gatekeeper policies controlling access to specialists have encountered resistance among consumers, who in a competitive environment could simply switch plans. Increased competency of general medical providers could alter patient preferences and facilitate shifting. Yet many general medical clinicians express a reluctance to treat more depressed patients and prefer to have the option of referral. Long-term reorientation of practice priorities would require redefining the clinician's role through education and training, which could take a generation to occur.

Improving cost-effectiveness does not mean lowering treatment costs, and we have little doubt that quality improvement within each specialty sector increases health care costs for that sector. In contrast, much of the discussion about coverage for mental health care reflects an implicit hope that higher quality care is the magic bullet that miraculously lowers overall health care costs, the so-called cost-offset effect. This wishful thinking appears to be so ingrained that our cost-effectiveness work is regularly misquoted as evidence for it— even though we explicitly say that quality improvement by itself raises treatment costs.

But even if the idea that health care plans can save money through better care is too simple-minded, and that the correct answer is that plans can reduce wasteful use of money, we would agree that cost offsets can exist from a larger societal perspective because the main component of the social costs of depression are indirect losses through morbidity, not direct treatment costs. Low treatment rates leading to prolonged morbidity may therefore be socially inefficient, and resources could be redistributed to make everybody better off. Unfortunately, the MOS was not designed to analyze social costs.

Policy Implications

We have not discussed the policy perspective of how socially efficient health care can be developed, but our research suggests that quality improvement for the care of depression is necessary to improve the value of care. In textbook economy, low-value products and services are not viable in the long-run, regardless of their price. Automobiles ranging from subcompact to luxury models are sold, but U.S. automobile manufacturers had to improve quality and cut prices to compete successfully against European and Asian manufacturers who simply provided better values. This gives some hope for care for depression, but market forces unfortunately are not always successful. There are two reasons markets may fail to make care for depression socially efficient: externalities and information problems.

High-quality care leading to better health outcomes creates benefits for many parties that are not involved in health care. Such positive externalities accrue to the employers of better-treated patients through reduced absenteeism and higher productivity; family members and friends through lower burdens of care for sick individuals; and government agencies through fewer transfer payments (welfare, unemployment, disability). But a health care plan has no obvious way to capture all of these indirect benefits and only shoulders the increased direct treatment costs of higher quality care, diminishing its financial incentives to improve quality of care. This implies that even under perfect information about health care benefits and costs of treatment, a purely market-based insurance system will not equate the social costs and social benefits that are central to an efficient system.

Externalities are not the worst problem under the current employment-based system, as most of the indirect economic benefits are likely to be obtained by patients and their employers, who are paying for health care and insurance. An even bigger problem may be imperfect information: employers cannot determine if a health care plan that claims to provide higher quality care is worth the additional expenditures. This is partly a problem of quality-of-care measurement and accountability of care and partly a problem of our ignorance about the indirect benefits of health care.

The policy implications are twofold: first, there must be incentives for higher quality care, ideally a reimbursement scheme that permits plans to capture their social contribution. Excluding or markedly limiting mental health care coverage seems inconsistent with that task, and a purely employment-based insurance may be insufficient. But good policy decisions in that area require more information on the potential for improving value of care, health outcomes, and cost implications across disease conditions that compete for resources.

Second, from a regulatory perspective, it is necessary to establish standard quality-of-care measurements that would allow higher quality providers to identify themselves convincingly as such. Plans and employers need more feedback on outcomes, costs, and value of care. We emphasize this broader outcomes framework, even though many plans are struggling with implementing basic outcomes measures and do not yet have the data or methods to identify this broader profile of impacts.

Toward Useful Evaluations of Depression Care

How can health care delivery systems and plans obtain better information about their performance? The availability of data alone does not assure an ability to use those data well. Suitable evaluation questions, design, and analytic capability are more important than selecting a particular health outcome or process measure.

Good data and analytic management capabilities are not cheap in terms of the necessary infrastructure to obtain data on outcomes or to clean, analyze, and interpret them, or in terms of opportunity costs (time taken from other activities) for providers, patients, and administrators. It does not seem wise to spend resources developing a system that is not adequately designed for addressing questions of interest, yet we repeatedly encounter costly activities that do not seem to add up to very much. We therefore emphasize the importance of clarifying which questions one wishes to answer, and then assuring that data collection, management systems, and analytic strategies are appropriate for answering those questions before spending hundreds of thousands or even millions of dollars.

The scope of questions has major implications for measurement, data collection, and analytic strategies. Internal comparisons to evaluate different management decisions are much more demanding than external comparisons that measure quality of care and outcomes against an external benchmark. Typical questions for internal comparisons focus on resource allocations and the accountability of a health care system, such as:

1. Do certain interventions benefit enrollees or patients in measurable ways?
2. Which types of expenditures have the strongest impacts and for whom?
3. What is the most cost-effective way of managing patients who pose very high financial risks to a health care delivery system?

4. When cheaper services are introduced, do patient outcomes suffer?
5. Is putting money into prevention programs versus improved direct clinical services more cost-effective?

These are very demanding questions, and one encounters numerous pitfalls in trying to analyze them. The MOS performed similar internal comparisons, and we discussed some generic design and analysis issues in Chapter 4. In observational studies, selection biases (casemix differences) are of particular importance, but other sampling issues also need to be anticipated: Are sample sizes large enough to detect effects reliably? Are clinically precise process indicators available? Are outcomes assessed independently of a visit to a provider? Strong designs can require substantial resources. For example, the larger MOS cost about $12 million including analyses, and the depression component about $4 million.

Most users of outcomes research are likely to settle for much simpler descriptive information for external comparisons, however, and such studies can be performed at a fraction of the costs. The tables in the appendixes provide an example of benchmark data for such comparisons. Other benchmark data are contained in clinical practice guidelines, which usually represent a normative ideal, based on a synthesis of scientific evidence and expert opinion. Typical questions for descriptive external comparisons are:

1. How do our enrollees or patients compare in sickness with similar persons across the nation?
2. How does our quality of care compare with other providers and with recommended practice?
3. Where are the most important areas for improving quality of care for depression?
4. Are outcomes comparable to what would be expected for depressed patients in similar health care delivery systems?

The key design issue for these questions is to identify an appropriate comparison data set (such as the MOS) and to adjust newly collected data (from a health care plan) to the patient characteristics for the standard data. Of course, usual-care data such as the MOS do not necessarily reflect acceptable quality-of-care standards.

Based on our experience with a large number of measures, we recommend a basic set of measures for depression that includes clinician detection, use of appropriate antidepressant medication, initially and over time, avoidance of regular minor tranquilizer use, occurrence of counseling for depression, continuity of plan participation and patient-provider relationship, and at least brief measures of morbidity outcomes. The SF-36 may be useful morbidity measures, but a simple count of serious limitations, which has high face validity and a direct interpretation, may be as useful with larger sample sizes. Patient satisfaction is commonly used as a proxy measure of quality of care, but patient satisfaction is affected by many factors other than the quality of clinical care and is not necessarily related to outcomes, although it may be useful in studies that cannot measure processes of care or health outcomes directly or as a predictor of disenrollment.

Clearly, we have a long way to go before research can provide information that is reliable and suitably comprehensive for addressing larger policy issues, and even further before the necessary data and analytic tools are widely available and appropriately used in public and private sector health care delivery systems. The MOS was a first step and established where quality problems are common, how crucial it is to consider health and cost outcomes simultaneously, and the value of a comprehensive overview or "systems diagnosis" of care for a tracer condition within a single study. Future studies need an even stronger integration of economic and clinical health services research in order to separate out the different effects of specific clinical processes, as well as the larger policies that influence these processes, on direct treatment and indirect social costs. Depression is only one of many illnesses that need to be studied from such a broad perspective. This book provides a conceptual model that can be adopted for larger policy studies and measures that can be used in less ambitious evaluations.

Appendixes
Notes
References
Index

Appendix A

Scoring Rules and Item Content for Health-Related Quality-of-Life Measures

The following pages present scoring rules for the health-related quality-of-life (HRQOL) measures presented in Chapter 5. Questionnaire items with their associated item numbers are given at the end of Appendix A. Measures are scored in a two-step process. First, Table A.1 shows how to recode response categories for each questionnaire item. The original response categories shown in column two are recoded to the values shown in column three. Most items, except those used to score serious limitations, sexual functioning, sleep problems, and physical/psychophysiologic symptoms, are scored so that a high score defines a more favorable health state. In addition, each item, except for those used to score serious limitations, is scored from 0 to 100. Second, Table A.2 shows which items are averaged together to create each HRQOL measure. For all measures, items that are missing are not taken into account when calculating the scale scores. Thus measures represent the average for all items in the scale that the respondent answers. The serious limitations measure, in contrast, is a count of number of limitations that can range from 0 to 4.

Table A.1   Step 1: Recoding Items

Item numbers	Change original response category	To recoded value of
9, 10	1 →	1
	2 →	0
1, 3, 4, 24a, 24d, 27a, 27d, 27e	1 →	100
	2 →	75
	3 →	50
	4 →	25
	5 →	0
6a,* 6b,* 6c, 6d, 6e, 6f,	1 →	0
6g, 6h, 6i, 6j	2 →	50
	3 →	100
7a, 7b, 7c, 7d, 8a, 8b, 8c	1 →	0
	2 →	100
2, 11b, 11c, 20, 23, 25b,	1 →	100
25c, 25d, 25e	2 →	80
	3 →	60
	4 →	40
	5 →	20
	6 →	0
11a, 11d, 13, 14, 15, 16,	1 →	0
17, 18, 19, 21, 22, 25a, 25f	2 →	20
	3 →	40
	4 →	60
	5 →	80
	6 →	100
5, 12a, 12b, 12c, 12d, 12e,	1 →	0
12f, 12g, 24b, 24c, 27b,	2 →	25
27c, 27f	3 →	50
	4 →	75
	5 →	100
26a, 26b, 26c, 26d, 26e	1 →	0
	2 →	33.33
	3 →	66.67
	4 →	100
	5 →	0

*Items 6a and 6b are coded as follows for the serious limitations measure: 1 or 2 = 1; 3 = 0.

Table A.2 Step 2: Averaging Items to Form Scales

Scale	Number of items	After recoding per Table A.1, average the following items
Physical functioning	10	6a, 6b, 6c, 6d, 6e, 6f, 6g, 6h, 6i, 6j
Serious limitations	4	(6a, 6b, 9, 10)[a]
Role–physical	4	7a, 7b, 7c, 7d
Role–emotional	3	8a, 8b, 8c
Bodily pain	2	2, 3
Mental health	5	19, 20, 21, 22, 23
Cognitive functioning	6	13, 14, 15, 16, 17, 18
Social functioning	2	4, 5
Sexual functioning	4	26a, 26b, 26c (26d, 26e)[b]
Marital functioning	6	27a, 27b, 27c, 27d, 27e, 27f
Energy/fatigue	4	11a, 11b, 11c, 11d
Sleep problems	6	25a, 25b, 25c, 25d, 25e, 25f
Physical/psychophysiologic symptoms	7	12a, 12b, 12c, 12d, 12e, 12f, 12g
General health perceptions	5	1, 24a, 24b, 24c, 24d

a. Count across each item so that the score ranges from 0 to 4.
b. Item 26d for men only; 26e for women only.

Health Outcomes Survey Items

1. In general, would you say your health is:

                                          (Circle one)

                        Excellent   1
                        Very good   2
                        Good   3
                        Fair   4
                        Poor   5

2. How much *bodily* pain have you generally had during the *past 4 weeks?*

                                          (Circle one)

                        None   1
                        Very mild   2
                        Mild   3
                        Moderate   4
                        Severe   5
                        Very severe   6

3. During the *past 4 weeks,* how much did pain interfere with your normal work (including both work outside the home and house-work)?

                                          (Circle one)

                        Not at all   1
                        A little bit   2
                        Moderately   3
                        Quite a bit   4
                        Extremely   5

4. During the *past 4 weeks*, to what extent has your physical health or emotional problems interfered with your normal social activities with family, friends, neighbors, or groups?

(Circle one)

Not at all	1
Slightly	2
Moderately	3
Quite a bit	4
Extremely	5

5. During the *past 4 weeks*, how much of the time has your *physical health* or *emotional problems* interfered with your social activities (like visiting with friends, relatives, etc.)?

(Circle one)

All of the time	1
Most of the time	2
Some of the time	3
A little of the time	4
None of the time	5

6. The following items are activities you might do during a typical day. *Does your health limit you* in these activities?

(Circle one number on each line)

Activities	Yes, limited a lot	Yes, limited a little	No, not limited at all
a. *Vigorous activities,* such as running, lifting heavy objects, participating in strenuous sports	1	2	3
b. *Moderate activities,* such as moving a table, pushing a vacuum cleaner, bowling, or playing golf	1	2	3
c. Lifting or carrying groceries	1	2	3
d. Climbing *several* flights of stairs	1	2	3
e. Climbing *one* flight of stairs	1	2	3
f. Bending, kneeling, or stooping	1	2	3
g. Walking *more than a mile*	1	2	3
h. Walking *several blocks*	1	2	3
i. Walking *one block*	1	2	3
j. Bathing or dressing yourself	1	2	3

7. During the *past 4 weeks*, have you had any of the following problems with your work or other regular daily activities *as a result of your physical health*? (Please answer Yes or No for each question.)

(Circle one number on each line)

	Yes	No
a. Cut down the *amount of time* you spent on work or other activities	1	2
b. *Accomplished less* than you would like	1	2
c. Were limited in the *kind* of work or other activities	1	2
d. Had *difficulty* performing the work or other activities (for example, it took extra effort)	1	2

8. During the *past 4 weeks*, have you had any of the following problems with your work or other regular daily activities *as a result of any emotional problems* (such as feeling depressed or anxious)? (Please answer Yes or No for each question.)

(Circle one number on each line)

	Yes	No
a. Cut down the *amount of time* you spent on work or other activities?	1	2
b. *Accomplished less* than you would like?	1	2
c. Didn't do work or other activities as *carefully* as usual?	1	2

9. Does your health *keep you* from working around the house?

(Circle one)

Yes	1
No	2

10. Does your health *keep you* from working at a paying job?

(Circle one)

Yes	1
No	2

11. How often during the *past 4 weeks* . . .

(Circle one number on each line)

	All of the time	Most of the time	A good bit of the time	Some of the time	A little of the time	None of the time
a. did you feel worn out?	1	2	3	4	5	6
b. did you have a lot of energy?	1	2	3	4	5	6
c. did you feel full of pep?	1	2	3	4	5	6
d. did you feel tired?	1	2	3	4	5	6

12. How often have you had any of the following symptoms during the *past 4 weeks?*

(Circle one number on each line)

	Never	Once or twice	A few times	Fairly often	Very often
a. Stiffness, pain, swelling or soreness of muscles or joints	1	2	3	4	5
b. Coughing that produced sputum	1	2	3	4	5
c. Backaches or lower back pains	1	2	3	4	5
d. Nausea (upset stomach)	1	2	3	4	5
e. Acid indigestion, heartburn, or feeling bloated after meals	1	2	3	4	5
f. Heavy feelings in arms and legs	1	2	3	4	5
g. Lump in throat	1	2	3	4	5

13. How much of the time, during the *past month*, did you have difficulty reasoning and solving problems; for example, making plans, making decisions, learning new things?

(Circle one)

All of the time	1
Most of the time	2
A good bit of the time	3
Some of the time	4
A little of the time	5
None of the time	6

14. During the *past month,* how much of the time did you have difficulty doing activities involving concentration and thinking?

(Circle one)

All of the time	1
Most of the time	2
A good bit of the time	3
Some of the time	4
A little of the time	5
None of the time	6

15. During the *past month*, how much of the time did you become confused and start several actions at a time?

(Circle one)

All of the time	1
Most of the time	2
A good bit of the time	3
Some of the time	4
A little of the time	5
None of the time	6

16. During the *past month*, how much of the time did you forget, for example, things that happened recently, where you put things, appointments?

(Circle one)

All of the time	1
Most of the time	2
A good bit of the time	3
Some of the time	4
A little of the time	5
None of the time	6

17. How much of the time, during the *past month*, did you have trouble keeping your attention on any activity for long?

(Circle one)

All of the time	1
Most of the time	2
A good bit of the time	3
Some of the time	4
A little of the time	5
None of the time	6

18. How much of the time, during the *past month*, did you react slowly to things that were said or done?

(Circle one)

All of the time	1
Most of the time	2
A good bit of the time	3
Some of the time	4
A little of the time	5
None of the time	6

19. How much of the time, during the *past month*, have you been a very nervous person?

(Circle one)

All of the time	1
Most of the time	2
A good bit of the time	3
Some of the time	4
A little of the time	5
None of the time	6

20. How much of the time, during the *past month*, have you felt calm and peaceful?

(Circle one)

All of the time	1
Most of the time	2
A good bit of the time	3
Some of the time	4
A little of the time	5
None of the time	6

21. How much of the time, during the *past month*, have you felt downhearted and blue?

(Circle one)

All of the time	1
Most of the time	2
A good bit of the time	3
Some of the time	4
A little of the time	5
None of the time	6

22. How much of the time, during the *past month*, have you felt so down in the dumps that nothing could cheer you up?

(Circle one)

All of the time	1
Most of the time	2
A good bit of the time	3
Some of the time	4
A little of the time	5
None of the time	6

23. During the *past month*, how much of the time have you been a happy person?

(Circle one)

All of the time	1
Most of the time	2
A good bit of the time	3
Some of the time	4
A little of the time	5
None of the time	6

24. How true or false is *each* of the following statements for you?

(Circle one number on each line)

	Definitely true	Mostly true	Don't know	Mostly false	Definitely false
a. I am as healthy as anybody I know	1	2	3	4	5
b. I seem to get sick a little easier than other people	1	2	3	4	5
c. I expect my health to get worse	1	2	3	4	5
d. My health is excellent	1	2	3	4	5

25. How often during the *past 4 weeks* did you . . .

(Circle one number on each line)

	All of the time	Most of the time	A good bit of the time	Some of the time	A little of the time	None of the time
a. get enough sleep to feel rested upon waking in the morning?	1	2	3	4	5	6
b. awaken short of breath or with a headache?	1	2	3	4	5	6
c. have trouble falling asleep?	1	2	3	4	5	6
d. awaken during your sleep time and have trouble falling asleep again?	1	2	3	4	5	6
e. have trouble staying awake during the day?	1	2	3	4	5	6
f. get the amount of sleep you needed?	1	2	3	4	5	6

26. These next questions are about the way health problems might interfere with your sex life. These questions are personal, but your answers are important in understanding how health problems affect people's lives.

How much of a problem was *each* of the following during the *past 4 weeks?*

(Circle one number on each line)

	Not a problem	Little bit of a problem	Somewhat of a problem	Very much a problem	Not applicable
a. Lack of sexual interest	1	2	3	4	5
b. Unable to relax and enjoy sex	1	2	3	4	5
c. Difficulty in becoming sexually aroused	1	2	3	4	5
Men Only d. Difficulty getting or keeping an erection	1	2	3	4	5
Women Only e. Difficulty in having an orgasm	1	2	3	4	5

27. The following statements are about your relationship with your spouse or partner. How true or false has *each* one been for you during the *past 4 weeks?* (If you do not have a spouse or partner, please answer these about the person you feel closest to.)

(Circle one number on each line)

	Definitely true	Mostly true	Don't know	Mostly false	Definitely false
a. We said anything we wanted to say to each other	1	2	3	4	5
b. We often had trouble sharing our personal feelings	1	2	3	4	5
c. It was hard to blow off steam with each other	1	2	3	4	5
d. I felt close to my spouse or partner	1	2	3	4	5
e. My spouse or partner was supportive of me	1	2	3	4	5
f. We tended to rely on other people for help rather than on each other	1	2	3	4	5

Scoring Rules and Item Content for Process of Clinical Care Measures

This appendix provides specific scoring rules and the actual items for the process measures described in Chapter 5. They are adapted from the full questionnaires completed by clinicians and patients participating in the MOS. We first provide this information for the twelve measures of clinical treatment of depression and then provide corresponding information for the seven measures of clinician usual style of care. At the end of this appendix, we provide scoring rules for the brief depression screener used in the MOS (Burnam et al., 1988).

Tables B.1 and B.2 give recoding rules for items used to score the clinical treatment of depression measures. Questionnaire items follow Table B.2. For example, questionnaire item 1 (Has this patient been depressed for a period of two weeks or more within the last year?) is used to create the "detection of depression" measure. If the clinician circles 1, 2, or 3 for item 1, the variable is coded "1"; otherwise, it is coded "0."

Measures of clinician usual counseling style are scored in a two-step process. Questionnaire items follow Tables B.3 and B.4. First, Table B.3 shows how to recode response categories for each questionnaire item. The original response categories shown in column two are recoded to the values shown in column three. Each item is scored on a scale of 0 to 100. Second, Table B.4 shows which items are averaged together to create each counseling style measure. For all measures, items that are missing are not taken into account when calculating the scale scores. Thus measures represent the average for all items in the scale that the respondent answers.

We would like to acknowledge additional MOS staff members who were responsible for developing some of these process measures. Sherrie

Kaplan, Ph.D., of the New England Medical Center developed the set of items designed to measure general interpersonal style (e.g., Participation Style and Shared Decision-Making). Marcia Daniels, M.D., a private practitioner in Los Angeles, contributed to the development of the counseling style measures.

Table B.1 Recoding Items[a]

Measure	Derived variable equals "1" if
Detection of depression	Q1 = 1, 2, or 3
Depression visit	Q2 = 1 or Q3 = 1
Mental health visit	(Q2 = 1 or 2) or (Q3 = 1 or Q4 = 1) or Q7 = 1
Psychosocial visit	(Q2 = 1, 2, or 3) or (Q3 = 1 or Q4 = 1 or Q5 = 1) or Q7 = 1
Counseling for depression	Q3 = 1
Used antidepressants	Q9 = a medication from column 1 in Table B.2
Effective use of antidepressants	Q9 = a medication from column 1 in Table B.2 and Q10 ≥ dosage in column 2 or column 3
Used minor tranquilizers	Q9 = a medication from column 4 in Table B.2
Unmet need for depression care	Q13 = 1 and Q18 = 2
Unmet need for psychosocial care	(Q13 = 1 and Q18 = 2) or (Q14 = 1 and Q19 = 2) or (Q15 = 1 and Q20 = 2) or (Q16 = 1 and Q21 = 2) or (Q17 = 1 and Q22 = 2)
Appropriate care for depression	(Q1 = 1, 2, or 3) or (Q2 = 1 or Q3 = 1)
Referral to mental health specialty	Q7 = 1

a. All measures are derived by recoding original items into discrete indicators where "1" indicates that the particular criteria were met and "0" indicates that the criteria were not met.

Table B.2   List of Antidepressants and Minor Tranquilizers for Use in Coding Measures

Antidepressant medication	Cutoff point for subtherapeutic total daily dosage of antidepressant (mg)[a] for elderly patients	Cutoff point for subtherapeutic total daily dosage of antidepressant (mg)[a] for nonelderly patients	Minor tranquilizer medication
Amitriptyline	75	100	Alprazolam
Amoxapine	75	100	Butabarbital
Desipramine	75	100	Chloral hydrate
Doxepin	75	100	Chlordiazepoxied
Imipramine	75	100	Clonazepam
Isocarboxazid	20	30	Clorazepate
Nomifensine	50	100	Diazepam
Nortriptyline	50	75	Diphenhydramine
Phenelzine	30	45	Flurazepam
Protriptyline	20	30	Hydroxyzine
Tranylcypromine	10	20	Lorazepam
Trazodone	75	100	Meprobamate
Trimipramine	75	100	Oxazepam
—			Phenobarbital
—			Prazepam
—			Promethazine
—			Temazepam
—			Triazolam

a. From Katon et al. (1992).

Clinical Treatment of Depression Items

Clinician Screener

Detection, Counseling, Appropriate Care, and Referral

1. Has this patient been *depressed* for a period of two weeks or more within the last year?

(Circle one)

Yes—I provide the majority of care	1
Yes—another physician or therapist provides the majority of care	2
Yes—not under care	3
Don't know	4
No	5

2. What was the *main* diagnosis or problem addressed in this visit?

(Circle one)

Depression	1
Schizophrenia	2
Other emotional/family problems	3

During this visit did you spend *three minutes or more* counseling this patient about each of the following?

(Circle one number on each line)

	Yes	No
3. Depression?	1	2
4. Anxiety?	1	2
5. Other emotional or family problems?	1	2

6. How long did you spend *face-to-face* with this patient?

(Circle one)

Less than 5 minutes	1
6–10 minutes	2
11–15 minutes	3
16–20 minutes	4
21–30 minutes	5
31–60 minutes	6
More than 60 minutes	7

7. During this visit did you make a referral or request a *mental health consult or therapy?*

(Circle one)

Yes	No
1	2

Patient Assessment Questionnaire

Quality and Use of Psychotropic Medications

Please look at the label or container for this medication to answer the questions below.

8. What is the name of this medication? (Name may be on label or container.)

    Write in name of medication: _____

9. Please refer to the Medications Code List printed on the inside of the back cover of this booklet and write in the code number listed for this drug. (Enter "999" if the medication does not appear on the code list.)

    Write in code number: ☐☐☐

10. In the space below, please copy the dosage of this medication exactly as it appears on the medication label, including any letters that follow the numbers (for example, 250 mg). If there is a decimal point, please be sure to include it (for example, .25 mg).

Write in the dosage on label: _____

Check box if no dosage listed ☐

11. During the past 30 days, on how many days did you actually take this medication? (If you haven't taken this medication in the last 30 days, write in "00.")

Write in number of days: ☐☐☐

12. When you actually take this medication, what is the total number of pills, capsules, measures of liquid, injections, or other measures of this medication that you usually take each day?

Write in number of pills, capsules, measures, or injections taken per day: _____

Unmet Need

During the past 6 months, did you feel you needed or wanted help for any of the following problems?

(Circle one number on each line)

	Yes	No
13. Feeling depressed or blue	1	2
14. Family or marital problems	1	2
15. Alcohol or drugs	1	2
16. Sexual problems or concerns	1	2
17. Other personal, emotional, behavioral, or mental problems	1	2

During the *past 6 months,* for which problems did you actually receive care?

(Circle one number on each line)

	Yes	No
18. Feeling depressed or blue	1	2
19. Family or marital problems	1	2
20. Alcohol or drugs	1	2
21. Sexual problems or concerns	1	2
22. Other personal, emotional, behavioral, or mental problems	1	2

Type of Counseling

23. What kind of mental health specialist did you see most often in the *past 6 months?*

(Circle one)

Psychiatrist	1
Psychologist	2
Psychiatric social worker	3
Psychiatric nurse	4
Marriage or family counselor	5
Other	6
Don't know	7

24. What kind of counseling or therapy did you receive *most often* in the *past 6 months?*

(Circle one)

Individual therapy	1
Group therapy	2
Family therapy	3
Other	4
None	5

Table B.3 Step 1: Recoding Items

Item numbers	Change original response category	To recoded value of
1, 2, 3, 4, 5, 6, 7, 8	1 →	0
	2 →	33.33
	3 →	66.67
	4 →	100
9	1 →	0
	2 →	0
	3 →	0
	4 →	100
10	a	a
15, 16, 18, 20, 21, 22	1 →	0
	2 →	25
	3 →	50
	4 →	75
	5 →	100
11, 12, 13, 14, 17, 19	1 →	100
	2 →	75
	3 →	50
	4 →	25
	5 →	0

a. Create one discrete indicator for each of the six response categories by coding a "100" if the response was circled and a "0" if the response was not circled.

Table B.4 Step 2: Averaging Items to Form Scales

Scale	Number of items	After recoding per Table B.3, average the following items:
Usual counseling style		
Initiative	4	1, 2, 3, 4
Perceived skill	4	5, 6, 7, 8
Intensity	1	9
Techniques	a	a
Preference for depression counseling	4	11, 12, 13, 14
Usual interpersonal style		
Egalitarian participation	4	16, 18, 20, 22
Share treatment decision-making	4	15, 17, 19, 21

a. Six dichotomous indicators, one for each of the six response categories, are created from item number 10.

Clinician Usual Counseling Style Items

Clinician Background Questionnaire

In the *last month*, what *usually* prompted you to discuss the following issues with your patients?

(Circle one number on each line)

	Did not discuss	Patient brought it up	I suspected a problem	Routinely discussed with all patients seen
1. Marital or family problems	1	2	3	4
2. Depression	1	2	3	4
3. Sexual functioning	1	2	3	4
4. Coping with physical illness or symptoms	1	2	3	4

How *skilled* do you think you are in counseling patients about the following issues?

(Circle one number on each line)

	Not at all skilled	Slightly skilled	Somewhat skilled	Very skilled
5. Marital or family problems	1	2	3	4
6. Depression	1	2	3	4
7. Sexual functioning	1	2	3	4
8. Coping with physical illness or symptoms	1	2	3	4

9. In the *last month*, when you dealt with emotional issues or patients' personal problems, how much time did you *usually* take?

(Circle one)

Did not deal with these issues at all	1
Used less than 5 minutes of an office visit	2
Used 5–10 minutes of an office visit	3
Used more than 10 minutes of an office visit	4

10. In the *last month*, which of the following techniques did you usually use in face-to-face counseling of your patients for personal, emotional, or family problems?

(Circle all that apply)

Education or advice	1
Interpretations of confrontations	2
Counseling family members	3
Behavioral treatments (e.g., relaxation or stress management)	4
Psychodynamic therapy	5
Did not personally counsel	6

For *each* of the following patient groups, how likely are you to provide ongoing (three or more visits) face-to-face counseling to treat moderate to severe depression?

(Circle one number on each line)

	Very likely	Somewhat likely	Unsure	Somewhat unlikely	Very unlikely
11. Depression, no major medical illness	1	2	3	4	5
12. Depression and recent myocardial infarction	1	2	3	4	5
13. Depression and hypertension	1	2	3	4	5
14. Depression and diabetes	1	2	3	4	5

Clinician Usual Interpersonal Style Items

Clinician Background Questionnaire

To what extent do you *agree* or *disagree* with the following statements?

On the line next to *each* statement, circle one number (from 1 to 5) for the opinion that is closest to your own.

(Circle one number on each line)

	Strongly agree	Agree	Neither agree nor disagree	Disagree	Strongly disagree
15. I prefer that patients leave decisions about their treatment up to me	1	2	3	4	5
16. Good doctors use their authority to shape patient behavior	1	2	3	4	5
17. If I make patients feel that they are making treatment choices themselves, their disease management is better	1	2	3	4	5
18. Treatment recommendations presented with authority are more likely to be accepted by patients	1	2	3	4	5
19. It is best to let patients participate in decisions whenever choices between treatment options are available	1	2	3	4	5

	Strongly agree	Agree	Neither agree nor disagree	Disagree	Strongly disagree
20. Among competent professionals, those who maintain a strong air of authority usually obtain the best results in treating patients	1	2	3	4	5
21. Most patients are unable to make intelligent choices about their care	1	2	3	4	5
22. Sometimes it is best to pressure patients to get them to do what is best for them	1	2	3	4	5

Brief Screener for Depression

The items in the patient screener (below) were used to screen for depression in the MOS. The screener was completed at the time of screening by patients visiting their providers. Table B.5 gives recoding rules for the eight items used to screen patients. After individual items are recoded as in Table B.5, formulas are presented that can be used to create a dichotomous indicator where "1" indicates high probability of current major depression, zero otherwise.

After scoring items as in Table B.5, the following procedures should be used to create the final dichotomous indicator. First, create a continuous score (prdep) using the following formulas:

$$prdep = 1/(1 + \exp(-pdscore))$$

where

$$pdscore = -6.543 + 1.078 \cdot Q3 + 0.329 \cdot Q4$$
$$- 0.280 \cdot Q5 - 0.269 \cdot Q6 + 0.185 \cdot Q7$$
$$+ 0.288 \cdot Q8 + 2.712 \cdot Q1 + 2.182 \cdot Q2.$$

Second, score patient as screening positive for depression (e.g., score of "1") if prdep is greater than 0.06. If prdep is missing, code patient as positive for depression if patient answered 1 to Question 1 or Question 2 and answered 1, 2, or 3 to Q3, Q4, Q5, Q6, Q7, or Q8 (after responses are recoded as in Table B.5).

Table B.5 Recoding of Items Used to Screen for Depression

Item numbers	Change original response category	To recoded value of
Q1, Q2	1	1
	2	0
Q3, Q4, Q5, Q7, Q8	1	0
	2	1
	3	2
	4	3
Q6	1	3
	2	2
	3	1
	4	0

Patient Screener

Q1. In the past year, have you had *2 weeks or more* during which you felt sad, blue, or depressed; or when you lost all interest or pleasure in things that you usually cared about or enjoyed?

(Circle one)

Yes	1
No	2

Q2. Have you felt depressed or sad much of the time in the *past year?*

(Circle one)

Yes	1
No	2

For *each statement* below, circle one number that *best* describes how much of the time you felt or behaved this way *during the past week.*

(Circle one number on each line)

During the Past Week:	Rarely or none of the time (less than one day)	Some or a little of the time (1–2 days)	Occasionally or a moderate amount of the time (3–4 days)	Most or all of the time (5–7 days)
Q3. I felt depressed	1	2	3	4
Q4. I had crying spells	1	2	3	4
Q5. I felt sad	1	2	3	4
Q6. I enjoyed life	1	2	3	4
Q7. My sleep was restless	1	2	3	4
Q8. I felt that people disliked me	1	2	3	4

Appendix C

Descriptive Statistics
for Outcome Measures

This appendix provides descriptive statistics for outcome measures. Tables C.1 and C.2 provide descriptive statistics for clinical measures by type of depression and by specialty of treating provider. Unadjusted means and percentages for clinical outcome measures show, as one would expect, that patients with current depressive disorder have more current symptoms of depression relative to persons with subthreshold depression, and the highest numbers of symptoms are reported for those with current double depression. Patients of psychiatrists and nonpsychiatric mental health specialists tend to be the most psychologically sick over time. They have more current symptoms of depression at baseline and are more likely to develop a new episode of depressive disorder over a two-year interval. Patients of psychiatrists also appear less likely to remit. This demonstrates that clinical status differences and prognosis are sufficiently different by specialty that outcome comparisons are only appropriate with careful stratification and adjustment for sickness differences.

Tables C.3–C.9 show characteristics of HRQOL measures by type of depression and specialty of treating provider. Mean HRQOL scores tend to be toward the sicker end (poorer functioning or well-being) for more severe forms of depression (current disorder and among those more chronic forms). Further, patients of psychiatrists also tend to have poorer functioning and well-being; but patients of general medical providers have the lowest levels of physical functioning. On some measures, sicker patients (and mental health specialty patients) are the most likely to have the worst possible health score. This means both that sicker patients have poorer HRQOL and that there is greater risk that the scales are not fully

188

capturing the HRQOL impact for sicker patients. The result is that conclusions about depression's impact on HRQOL for sicker patients are conservative.

Table C.10 shows change in HRQOL outcomes over two years by type of depression. For all but four scales (serious limitations, sexual functioning, sleep problems, physical symptoms), an increase (more positive change score) over time indicates improved health. Patients with current depressive disorder at baseline changed much more than did those with subthreshold depression.

We used a factor analysis to confirm that the two-factor model of health status applies among depressed patients. Table C.11 presents the results (rotated factor loadings using an oblique rotation method) separately by type of depression. We excluded serious limitations, which has overlapping items with other measures. For each type of depression except double depression, the two-factor solution is supported; but relative to all MOS patients with chronic medical conditions or depression, measures are more fully differentiated into either mental or physical health, especially for subthreshold patients. For example, social functioning and marital problems load with the mental health factor for all groups, and this finding is consistent with the emphasis in clinical studies of depressed patients on social functioning outcomes. It is not surprising that sleep is a mental health construct in depressed patients, given that sleep problems are primary symptoms of depression. But physical symptoms (including psychophysiologic symptoms) and to some extent general health perceptions emerge as more distinctly physical health domains in depressed patients than among all MOS patients.

For double depression, a single-factor solution is supported, probably because these patients are sick across all domains. Thus studies focusing exclusively on patients with double depression could include fewer HRQOL measures, as they are not distinct in this group.

Table C.12 gives correlations among HRQOL measures. As expected, different measures of mental health are more highly correlated with one another than with measures of physical health and vice versa. For example, correlations between physical functioning and other physical health measures are 0.56 for role–physical and 0.57 for bodily pain, compared with only 0.20 for role–emotional and 0.15 for mental health. In contrast, the correlation between mental health and role–emotional is 0.56. Health domains that were hypothesized to be correlated with both mental and physical health have moderate correlations with measures from each of these groupings. For example, the sleep problems measure has a correlation with physical functioning of -0.36 and with mental health of -0.47. The high associations of serious limitations with role–physical and physical functioning are due to overlapping items. This pattern of correlations supports all these domains as measures of health status, that is, interscale correlations are all at least moderate.

Table C.1 Descriptive Statistics for Clinical Measures by Type of Depression

Clinical measures	Subthreshold		Current major depression		Current dysthymia		Current double depression		Total	
	Mean	SD	Mean	SD	Mean	SD	Mean	SD	Mean	SD
Current symptoms (mean)	6.5	5.6	13.6[a]	5.1	13.1[a]	5.1	17.0	4.6	9.4	6.7
New episode (%)	32	47	—	—	52	50	—	—	38	48
Remission (%)	—	—	61	49	—	—	46	50	54	50

a. Means in a row with the same superscript do not differ significantly from one another at $p < .05$ or less.

Table C.2   Descriptive Statistics for Clinical Measures by Specialty of
Treating Provider

Clinical measures	General medical $\bar{X}$ (%)	SD	Psychiatrist $\bar{X}$ (%)	SD	Other mental health specialist $\bar{X}$ (%)	SD
Current symptoms (mean)	7.9	6.1	13.5	7.3	11.2	5.9
New episode (%)	28	45	48[a]	50	48[a]	50
Remission (%)	60[a]	49	36	48	60[a]	49

a. Means in a row with the same superscript do not differ significantly from one
another at $p < 0.05$ or less.

Table C.3 Characteristics of HRQOL Measures for Patients with Subthreshold Depression

Measure	No. of items	Mean	SD	Reliability	Item-total correlations	Floor (%)	Ceiling (%)	Complete data (%)
Physical functioning (+)[a]	10	73.2[c]	27.9	.94	.52–.85	1	24	89
Serious limitations (−)	4	1.3[c, d]	1.2	.72	.41–.70	31	5	—
Role–physical (+)	4	54.4[c, d]	38.9	.85	.64–.74	22	32	93
Role–emotional (+)	3	51.8[b, d]	40.4	.78	.59–.68	26	35	95
Bodily pain (+)	2	62.2[c, d]	22.3	.76	.62	1	18	94
Mental health (+)	5	62.6[b, c, d]	19.0	.85	.52–.74	<1	<1	92
Cognitive functioning (+)	6	77.3[b, c, d]	16.3	.86	.52–.74	0	9	90
Social functioning (+)	2	73.9[b, c, d]	25.1	.83	.71	<1	30	95
Sexual functioning (−)	5	26.4[b, c, d]	31.7	.88	.63–.83	40	6	88
Marital functioning (+)	6	65.2[b, d]	20.7	.78	.34–.68	<1	4	85
Energy/fatigue (+)	4	49.5[b, c, d]	20.4	.82	.60–.70	1	0	94
Sleep problems (−)	6	33.9[b, c, d]	19.0	.79	.41–.63	<1	0	92
Physical/psychophysiologic symptoms (−)	7	26.4[c, d]	17.4	.67	.22–.50	2	0	88
General health perceptions (+)	5	57.9[c, d]	20.5	.75	.33–.72	<1	<1	92

Note: Floor = lowest possible score; ceiling = highest possible score.

a. A (+) high score indicates better health; a (−) high score indicates worse health.

b. Mean is significantly different from mean of patients with current major depression at $p < .05$ or less.

c. Mean is significantly different from mean of patients with dysthymia at $p < .05$ or less.

d. Mean is significantly different from mean of patients with double depression at $p < .05$ or less.

Table C.4 Characteristics of HRQOL Measures for Patients with Current Major Depression

Measure	No. of items	Mean	SD	Reliability	Item-total correlations	Floor (%)	Ceiling (%)	Complete data (%)
Physical functioning (+)[a]	10	78.1[c]	24.7	.93	.59–.81	<1	29	91
Serious limitations (−)	4	1.5[c]	1.2	.72	.31–.70	29	4	—
Role–physical (+)	4	48.8	40.3	.87	.68–.75	30	27	97
Role–emotional (+)	3	42.1[d]	41.0	.81	.56–.74	39	26	97
Bodily pain (+)	2	59.2[c]	23.6	.80	.67	<1	14	94
Mental health (+)	5	50.3[d]	20.8	.86	.43–.78	0	0	93
Cognitive functioning (+)	6	69.5[d]	18.6	.87	.52–.77	0	4	90
Social functioning (+)	2	64.2[d]	27.4	.86	.76	2	24	94
Sexual functioning (−)	5	40.3	34.5	.89	.64–.85	24	10	92
Marital functioning (+)	6	55.3	26.6	.84	.24–.75	1	2	89
Energy/fatigue (+)	4	43.4[d]	22.2	.90	.76–.80	2	2	96
Sleep problems (−)	6	38.9[d]	18.1	.77	.33–.63	0	0	97
Physical/psychophysiologic symptoms (−)	7	28.9[c,d]	17.1	.72	.28–.55	4	0	92
General health perceptions (+)	5	56.1[c,d]	22.1	.77	.32–.76	0	3	94

Note: Floor = lowest possible score; ceiling = highest possible score.
a. A (+) high score indicates better health; a (−) high score indicates worse health.
c. Mean is significantly different from mean of patients with dysthymia at $p < .05$ or less.
d. Mean is significantly different from mean of patients with double depression at $p < .05$ or less.

Table C.5 Characteristics of HRQOL Measures for Patients with Current Dysthymia

Measure	No. of items	Mean	SD	Reliability	Item-total correlations	Floor (%)	Ceiling (%)	Complete data (%)
Physical functioning (+)[a]	10	63.0	30.0	.94	.51–.85	1	16	86
Serious limitations (−)	4	1.9	1.4	.79	.49–.83	25	12	—
Role–physical (+)	4	37.5	39.1	.81	.59–.71	42	20	91
Role–emotional (+)	3	41.1	41.4	.82	.59–.73	42	26	94
Bodily pain (+)	2	50.1	24.9	.80	.66	6	10	92
Mental health (+)	5	46.4[d]	19.9	.86	.59–.77	2	3	92
Cognitive functioning (+)	6	67.0[d]	19.8	.90	.65–.84	0	4	90
Social functioning (+)	2	56.2	25.7	.81	.69	2	8	94
Sexual functioning (−)	5	50.8	38.6	.88	.63–.80	24	17	86
Marital functioning (+)	6	59.3	26.7	.86	.42–.76	4	7	86
Energy/fatigue (+)	4	38.3	20.1	.79	.54–.65	<1	0	96
Sleep problems (−)	6	42.0	21.3	.76	.26–.64	<1	0	98
Physical/psychophysiologic symptoms (−)	7	37.0	19.2	.72	.26–.53	2	0	87
General health perceptions (+)	5	48.7	23.5	.78	.40–.74	0	0	94

Note: Floor = lowest possible score; ceiling = highest possible score.
a. A (+) high score indicates better health; a (−) high score indicates worse health.
d. Mean is significantly different from mean of patients with double depression at $p < .05$ or less.

Table C.6 Characteristics of HRQOL Measures for Patients with Current Double Depression

Measure	No. of items	Mean	SD	Reliability	Item-total correlations	Floor (%)	Ceiling (%)	Complete data (%)
Physical functioning (+)[a]	10	70.6	27.0	.90	.49–.76	0	22	89
Serious limitations (−)	4	1.8	1.3	.72	.43–.64	19	13	—
Role–physical (+)	4	41.2	37.4	.85	.61–.74	34	18	97
Role–emotional (+)	3	27.9	33.1	.67	.41–.61	48	10	97
Bodily pain (+)	2	54.3	25.3	.78	.64	3	14	96
Mental health (+)	5	37.9	18.5	.84	.52–.78	0	0	89
Cognitive functioning (+)	6	59.2	21.5	.88	.59–.77	0	<1	90
Social functioning (+)	2	49.2	28.1	.81	.68	8	5	95
Sexual functioning (−)	5	44.2	39.2	.89	.69–.80	31	15	91
Marital functioning (+)	6	54.3	26.1	.88	.56–.76	<1	3	80
Energy/fatigue (+)	4	34.0	18.4	.85	.67–.71	3	0	92
Sleep problems (−)	6	45.7	20.4	.76	.37–.62	0	<1	93
Physical/psychophysiologic symptoms (−)	7	37.6	20.5	.70	.24–.52	2	0	94
General health perceptions (+)	5	49.8	22.9	.76	.23–.72	3	0	91

Note: Floor = lowest possible score; ceiling = highest possible score.
a. A (+) high score indicates better health; a (−) high score indicates worse health.

Table C.7 Characteristics of HRQOL Measures for Depressed Patients of General Medical Specialists

Measure	No. of items	Mean	SD	Reliability	Item-total correlations	Floor (%)	Ceiling (%)	Complete data (%)
Physical functioning (+)[a]	10	67.5[b, c]	30.0	.94	.52–.83	1	22	88
Serious limitations (−)	4	1.6	1.3	.74	.45–.70	28	8	—
Role–physical (+)	4	49.3	40.1	.85	.66–.73	29	29	93
Role–emotional (+)	3	51.2[b, c]	40.7	.78	.56–.66	28	34	95
Bodily pain (+)	2	58.7	24.2	.78	.64	3	16	94
Mental health (+)	5	58.7[b]	20.8	.86	.52–.77	<1	1	91
Cognitive functioning (+)	6	74.7[b]	17.7	.87	.57–.75	0	8	90
Social functioning (+)	2	70.3[b, c]	26.6	.81	.68	2	26	94
Sexual functioning (−)	5	29.3[b]	33.8	.88	.61–.84	40	8	87
Marital functioning (+)	6	62.6	22.7	.82	.33–.69	<1	4	84
Energy/fatigue (+)	4	46.4	21.6	.85	.66–.72	2	<1	93
Sleep problems (−)	6	37.2	20.0	.80	.41–.65	<1	<1	93
Physical/psychophysiologic symptoms (−)	7	29.7	18.8	.70	.25–.52	3	0	88
General health perceptions (+)	5	53.6[c]	21.7	.76	.33–.71	1	<1	92

Note: Floor = lowest possible score; ceiling = highest possible score.

a. A (+) high score indicates better health; a (−) high score indicates worse health.

b. Mean is significantly different from patients of psychiatrists at $p < .05$ or less.

c. Mean is significantly different from patients of nonpsychiatric mental health specialists at $p < .05$ or less.

Table C.8 Characteristics of HRQOL Measures for Depressed Patients of Psychiatrists

Measure	No. of items	Mean	SD	Reliability	Item-total correlations	Floor (%)	Ceiling (%)	Complete data (%)
Physical functioning (+)[a]	10	79.0	23.1	.91	.55–.79	0	26	92
Serious limitations (−)	4	1.4[c]	1.2	.74	.46–.70	32	5	—
Role–physical (+)	4	52.9	38.4	.86	.62–.79	20	30	98
Role–emotional (+)	3	36.6	40.8	.85	.60–.81	45	25	98
Bodily pain (+)	2	61.8	23.0	.80	.67	<1	18	98
Mental health (+)	5	47.9[c]	22.6	.91	.59–.86	2	0	94
Cognitive functioning (+)	6	67.0[c]	23.1	.91	.64–.82	0	6	92
Social functioning (+)	2	61.8	30.9	.92	.86	4	22	96
Sexual functioning (−)	5	43.0	38.6	.91	.78–.83	25	16	92
Marital functioning (+)	6	61.0	23.6	.85	.51–.76	1	2	86
Energy/fatigue (+)	4	43.0	20.8	.87	.67–.77	<1	0	97
Sleep problems (−)	6	34.4	18.6	.76	.30–.61	0	0	94
Physical/psychophysiologic symptoms (−)	7	28.4	18.2	.65	.23–.48	2	0	90
General health perceptions (+)	5	57.4	22.7	.78	.35–.76	<1	<1	92

Note: Floor = lowest possible score; ceiling = highest possible score.
a. A (+) high score indicates better health; a (−) high score indicates worse health.
c. Mean is significantly different from patients of nonpsychiatric mental health specialists at $p < .05$ or less.

Table C.9 Characteristics of HRQOL Measures for Depressed Patients of Other Mental Health Specialists

Measure	No. of items	Mean	SD	Reliability	Item-total correlations	Floor (%)	Ceiling (%)	Complete data (%)
Physical functioning (+)[a]	10	83.6	17.6	.86	.40–.75	0	26	91
Serious limitations (−)	4	1.2	1.1	.64	.30–.61	29	3	—
Role–physical (+)	4	50.9	37.8	.83	.56–.73	22	26	96
Role–emotional (+)	3	39.1	37.1	.76	.53–.69	34	19	98
Bodily pain (+)	2	60.2	21.1	.77	.63	<1	14	92
Mental health (+)	5	55.4	19.7	.85	.45–.75	0	<1	90
Cognitive functioning (+)	6	72.9	16.9	.89	.57–.82	0	5	88
Social functioning (+)	2	64.0	24.7	.84	.73	<1	17	96
Sexual functioning (−)	5	36.6	34.4	.86	.63–.77	27	4	95
Marital functioning (+)	6	61.2	25.1	.86	.45–.75	3	5	88
Energy/fatigue (+)	4	45.4	19.8	.83	.53–.72	0	0	96
Sleep problems (−)	6	37.8	20.6	.74	.36–.56	<1	0	96
Physical/psychophysiologic symptoms (−)	7	28.8	18.1	.69	.25–.52	1	0	93
General health perceptions (+)	5	61.5	19.2	.73	.28–.66	0	<1	96

Note: Floor = lowest possible score; ceiling = highest possible score.
a. A (+) high score indicates better health; a (−) high score indicates worse health.

Table C.10 Change in HRQOL Outcomes over Two Years

	Subthreshold depression		Current major depression		Current dysthymia		Current double depression	
	$\bar{x}$	SD	$\bar{x}$	SD	$\bar{x}$	SD	$\bar{x}$	SD
Physical functioning	0.42	18.9	0.63	16.8	2.13	25.1	4.82	21.0
Serious limitations[a]	-0.12	1.1	-0.15	0.9	-0.24	1.4	-0.22	1.3
Role–physical	0.87	39.6	6.25	44.4	15.73	38.4	10.20	42.0
Role–emotional	7.24	44.3	22.91	53.8	4.34	46.0	16.40	45.0
Bodily pain	-0.41	18.9	0.43	20.8	5.26	28.2	5.43	22.7
Mental health	1.08	17.3	8.72	20.7	9.09	23.5	10.86	19.7
Cognitive functioning	-0.89	15.8	4.34	18.5	1.57	24.4	5.51	19.2
Social functioning	1.39	27.1	5.58	26.8	11.04	27.7	12.51	26.2
Sexual functioning[a]	-1.36	28.7	-6.21	32.9	-10.72	36.8	-10.90	33.2
Mental functioning	-0.55	25.2	3.76	24.5	3.90	22.9	3.91	22.0
Energy/fatigue	4.81	20.2	7.79	21.0	10.88	24.0	14.57	19.0
Sleep problems[a]	-2.23	17.8	-5.08	16.3	-1.66	25.7	-6.92	16.5
Physical/psychophysiologic symptoms[a]	1.89	17.3	-0.36	16.1	-1.94	18.6	-4.56	17.9
General health perceptions	2.90	19.8	3.79	17.9	4.12	22.4	5.80	18.7

a. A decrease over time indicates better outcomes for these measures.

Table C.11 Rotated Factor Loadings for Thirteen Functioning and Well-Being Measures

| | Type of depression | | | | | | | |
| | Subthreshold | | Current major depression | | Current dysthymia | | Current double depression | |
	Men.[a]	Phy.[b]	Men.	Phy.	Men.	Phy.	Men.	Phy.
Physical functioning	—[c]	.70	—	.73	—	.62	.55	.55
Role–physical	—	.64	—	.63	-.46	.53	.44	.49
Bodily pain	—	.69	—	.75	—	.79	.63	.52
Mental health	-.86	—	-.88	—	-.91	—	.70	—
Role–emotional	-.67	—	-.77	—	-.63	—	.53	—
Cognitive functioning	-.78	—	-.75	—	-.79	—	.74	—
Social functioning	-.61	—	-.70	—	-.74	—	.72	—
Symptoms	—	-.55	—	-.65	—	-.70	-.64	-.40
Energy/fatigue	-.50	.37	-.48	.46	-.59	.37	.56	—
Sleep problems	.49	—	.54	—	—	-.51	-.55	—
Health perceptions	—	.53	—	.57	-.41	.55	.52	.32
Sexual functioning	.29	—	.24	—	.41	—	-.45	—
Marital functioning	-.42	—	-.35	—	-.58	—	.20	-.19

a. Men. = mental health factor.
b. Phy. = physical health factor.
c. Secondary loadings less than 0.30 are omitted.

Table C.12 Correlations among Functioning, Well-Being, and Satisfaction at Baseline

		pfi	fstat	rolep	rolem	eft	mhi	scact	pain
Physical functioning (+)[a]	(pfi)	—							
Serious limitations (−)	(fstat)	-0.78	—						
Role–physical (+)	(rolep)	0.56	-0.60	—					
Role–emotional (+)	(rolem)	0.20	-0.28	0.42	—				
Energy/fatigue (+)	(eft)	0.45	-0.49	0.51	0.44	—			
Mental health (+)	(mhi)	0.15	-0.25	0.26	0.56	0.52	—		
Social functioning (+)	(scact)	0.40	-0.42	0.48	0.52	0.54	0.63	—	
Bodily pain (+)	(pain)	0.57	-0.54	0.60	0.25	0.47	0.28	0.47	—
Health perceptions (+)	(ghp)	0.56	-0.57	0.50	0.30	0.54	0.34	0.43	0.51
Cognitive functioning (+)	(cog)	0.21	-0.26	0.28	0.53	0.43	0.68	0.57	0.29
Marital functioning (+)	(famfnc)	0.01	-0.08	0.12	0.19	0.15	0.37	0.24	0.09
Sleep problems (−)	(slp)	-0.36	0.38	-0.40	-0.37	-0.52	-0.47	-0.47	-0.45
Psychophysiologic symptoms (−)	(sym)	-0.52	0.54	-0.54	-0.28	-0.46	-0.31	-0.42	-0.62
Sexual problems (−)	(sexprb)	-0.11	0.18	-0.21	-0.22	-0.24	-0.31	-0.26	-0.18

	ghp	cog	famfnc	slp	sym	sexprb
Physical functioning (+)[a] (pfi)						
Serious limitations (+) (fstat)						
Role–physical (+) (rolep)						
Role–emotional (+) (rolem)						
Energy/fatigue (+) (eft)						
Mental health (+) (mhi)						
Social functioning (+) (scact)						
Bodily pain (+) (pain)						
Health perceptions (+) (ghp)	—					
Cognitive functioning (+) (cog)	0.31	—				
Marital functioning (+) (famfnc)	0.11	0.30	—			
Sleep problems (−) (slp)	−0.40	−0.46	−0.19	—		
Psychophysiologic symptoms (−) (sym)	−0.49	−0.38	−0.11	0.47	—	
Sexual problems (−) (sexprb)	−0.19	−0.30	−0.21	0.19	0.20	—

a. A (+) high score indicates better health; a (−) high score indicates worse health.

Notes

2. Depression and Its Treatment

1. For an example of this controversy, see the discussions in Mirowsky and Ross, 1989; Swarz, Carroll, and Blazer, 1989; and Tweed and George, 1989.

2. For fuller descriptions of clinical features and course of major depression, see Keller, Lavori, Lewis, and Klerman, 1983; Keller et al., 1982; Klein et al., 1988; Kupfer, 1991; Sargeant et al., 1990; and Swindle, Cronkite, and Moos, 1989.

3. Dysthymia is a term developed for DSM-III and continued in DSM-IV, but other diagnostic schemes use labels such as chronic depression, chronic intermittent depression, minor depression, and so on. The heterogeneity in definitions across classification schemes for chronic depression has made it difficult to ascertain the applicability of studies of chronic depression, using other classifications, to DSM-III- or DSM-IV-defined dysthymia.

4. Norepinephrine is concentrated in areas of the brainstem that are involved in alertness, arousal, anxiety, and connections with the limbic system and hypothalamus, which regulate many emotions including pleasure. Serotonin is concentrated in areas of the midbrain, hypothalamus, and limbic system that regulate mood, sleep cycles, and appetite (Gitlin, 1990). Proposed abnormalities include reduced transmission, hypersensitivity of postsynaptic receptors with a compensatory reduction in transmission, and an imbalance in activity between norepinephrine-related (catecholamine) and serotonin-related (indoleamine) pathways (Caldecott-Hazard, Guze, et al., 1991; Mann, 1989).

5. For example, dexamethasone suppresses cortisol secretion in nondepressed persons but not in some forms of major depression, and a specific dexamethasone suppression test has been used in research studies to diagnose major depression and monitor treatment response. But as 50 percent of

depressed patients have a normal suppression response, and various other conditions and medications cause nonsuppression, the test has limited clinical utility.

6. Twin studies suggest a genetic pattern of transmission of more severe forms of major depression but are not conclusive because of the small samples; adoption studies suggest genetic factors for suicides but otherwise yield conflicting data about unipolar depression (Nurnberger and Gershon, 1992; Wender et al., 1986).

7. Although use of antidepressant medication is generally higher in mental health specialty practices, Olfson and Klerman (1992) found that among patients with diagnosed (that is, recognized) depression, the general medical sector had higher rates of use.

3. The Social Role of Depression and Health Care Policy

1. The ECA evaluated DSM-III disorders in adults aged eighteen and older in five U.S. sites cross-sectionally and longitudinally, using the Diagnostic Interview Schedule (DIS). The NCS assessed DSM-IIIR (revised) disorders in a nationally representative cross-sectional sample of persons aged fourteen to fifty-five, using the University of Michigan's version of the Composite International Diagnostic Interview (UM-CIDI).

2. Discrepancies between ECA and NCS rates are currently the subject of scientific debate, and could be due to the younger population for the NCS or methods effects such as differences in diagnostic criteria, sampling, instruments, or survey methods.

3. The rate drops to 17 percent if one includes other mental health specialists, such as psychologists and other nonphysician therapists (Myers et al., 1984; Weissman, Myers, and Thompson, 1981). In the ECA, 23 percent of persons with affective disorders received specialty mental health care in a year and 22 percent received some mental health care from a general medical clinician (Regier et al., 1993).

4. Studies indicate the following: middle-aged women who have high depression scores are less likely to work or participate in the labor force than their healthier counterparts, but this has only a minor economy-wide effect (Ruhm, 1992); mental health appears to be an important factor determining the labor force participation of older workers (Mitchell and Anderson, 1989); life cycle effects are important through educational attainment and occupational choice, at least in the case of alcoholism (Mullahy and Sindelar, 1993); and more than one in ten Social Security beneficiaries first entitled to Disability Insurance suffers from a mental or nervous disorder (Hennessey and Dykacs, 1989).

5. Some studies found that mental health specialists treat more serious psychiatric illnesses (Leaf et al., 1988; Greenley, Mechanic, and Cleary, 1987; Mechanic, Angel, and Davies, 1991; Sireling et al., 1985), whereas others found no differences between mental health specialty and general medical patients in the severity of major depression (Cooper-Patrick, Crum, and Ford, 1994; Coulehan et al., 1988) or psychological distress among mental health care users (Frank and Kamlet, 1990; Wells et al., 1987).

4. Evaluating Health Care Systems

1. The fundamental assumption of least-squares estimation (regression analysis and ANOVA) is that outcomes y are a linear function of the explanatory variables X and unobserved ("error") components ϵ, and that there is no correlation between the explanatory variables and the "error" term, mathematically $y = X\beta + \epsilon$ (1) and $E(X\epsilon) = 0$ (2). The estimate of β is calculated from the equation $\beta = (X'X)^{-1}X'y$ (3).

One selection problem may be that outcomes are more likely to be missing for individuals who did not receive treatment. In that case, the estimates from (3) will be biased. One correction approach is to estimate a probit selection equation and append a transformation of its predicted value (the estimated hazard or the inverse Mills ratio) as an additional regressor in the original regression equation (Amemiya, 1985). The validity of this approach rests on assumptions about the "error" distribution, but there have been recent nonparametric generalizations (Heckman, 1990).

2. To illustrate the instrumental variable technique in a selection problem resulting from missing information, consider a two-variable model in which outcomes are influenced by appropriate treatment (T) and casemix (C). We are interested in estimating the effectiveness of appropriate treatment in an observational study, but casemix is not fully observable. We expect (or know), however, that sicker patients are more likely to receive treatment. The correct model would be $y = T\beta_1 + C\beta_2 + \epsilon$, but the analyst estimates $y = T\beta_1{}^* + \epsilon^*$ (4). The expected value of this estimate is not the effectiveness of treatment β_1, but biased

$$E(\beta_1{}^*) = \beta_1 + \beta_2 \frac{\text{Cov }(T, C)}{\text{Var }(T)}.$$

This bias is caused by a violation of assumption (2) in note 1 of this chapter because $E(T\epsilon^*)$ is not zero.

The instrumental variable technique can obtain consistent estimates of β_1. It requires a variable (or set of variables) Z that is correlated with the variable of interest (T) but not with the omitted variables (casemix, or ϵ^*). Then the modification of (3) [note 1 of this chapter] $\beta_{IV} = (Z'X)^{-1}Z'y$ will yield consistent estimates of the structural parameters. This generalizes to more variables. For example, casemix is a multidimensional problem. If none of those variables are observed, we can expect that the bias is very strong and there may be little we can learn about the effectiveness of appropriate care from estimating (4). If we have good measures of casemix and include them in the regression, the selection bias caused by remaining unmeasured differences is likely to be minor. But as the bias cannot be determined, instrumental variables can be useful even with a measurement framework for casemix as extensive as the MOS.

3. One common misunderstanding regarding sensitivity tests comparing level and change analyses is the following: a linear regression of the change in outcomes (y_1-y_0) as the dependent variable on the baseline values of the variable that is differenced on the right-hand side (y_0) and other variables (x) provides exactly the same coefficients on those other variables as regressing the end level (y_1) on starting values (y_0) and other variables (x). This is not a test of the robustness of the model and the effect of confounding factors.

One occasionally hears the misleading claim that such differencing between baseline and follow-up removes the effect of sickness differences because "each patient serves as his or her own control." Differencing can remove constant individual-specific factors, but this clearly is not a valid argument here, as initial sickness also affects the rate of change in health status.

4. It is important to remember that the MOS did not measure all aspects equally well. Its strength was health status assessment, which avoids unobserved selection biases resulting from health status. Its weakness was economic measurement and analyzing issues in which selection according to economic factors is likely to be important, such as the relationship between health care utilization and payment switching; in this case, we did find evidence of selection bias that could not be controlled by variables collected in the MOS.

5. The criteria for a health condition to be a good tracer condition, adapted from Kessner, Kalk, and Singer (1973), are: (1) it is a common condition; (2) it can be defined precisely; (3) cases can be readily identified; (4) its severity can be defined and measured; (5) there are proven efficacious treatments (or prevention strategies) for the condition; (6) treatment varies considerably across alternative settings; (7) if factors other than treatment affect outcomes, they are known and measurable; and (8) the course of the condition is well understood.

6. These techniques assume that the two conditions $y = X\beta + \epsilon$ (1) and $E(X\epsilon) = 0$ (2) in the linear model and its analogues in nonlinear models are correct. In contrast, the selection problem is concerned with violations of the fundamental assumption (2). The nonparametric method relies on the fact

that standard models (such as linear regression or logistic regression maximum likelihood) continue to produce consistent and asymptotically normal parameter estimates under certain conditions and corrects the inconsistency of variance using what is called "robust standard errors," "sandwich variance estimator," or "Huber correction" (Fitzmaurice, Laird, and Rotnitzky, 1993; Huber, 1967; Liang and Zeger, 1986; Neuhaus, 1992; White, 1982). This approach to longitudinal data considers clustering effects or time dependence between responses mainly as a nuisance characteristic of the data (Fitzmaurice, Laird, and Rotnitzky, 1993). Nevertheless, this focus on marginal expectations and the nonparametric adjustment is not always the most efficient approach and does not take advantage of the longitudinal characteristics of the data. Panel data models, including fixed and random effects and coefficient models, can often be more appropriate (Bryk and Raudenbush, 1992; Chamberlain, 1984; Hsiao, 1986). These methods have only recently been discussed specifically in the mental health literature (Gibbons et al., 1993) but are likely to play a major role in future research.

5. Measuring Quality of Care and Outcomes

1. Data on psychotropic medication use were also obtained in a computer-assisted telephone interview at one- and two-year follow-ups. Patients described medications used in the last thirty days, or for at least one month since the last telephone assessment (about a one-year prior). Patients provided names, start- and end-dates of use, and, if used in the prior three months, typical total daily dosage.

2. We had a similar measure of preference for antidepressant medication, but we do not include it because correspondence was poor between this measure and patient medication use (Meredith, Wells, and Camp, 1994).

3. There are a number of different types of reliability (for example, internal consistency, test-retest, inter-rater reliability) that assess reliability and random error in different ways (for example, consistency of information across items, over time, or among different raters).

4. There are different ways to study validity (for example, types of validity include face, content, discriminant, convergent, predictive, criterion, known-groups validity, and a number of others) that have been defined in detail elsewhere (Stewart, 1990; Stewart, Hays, and Ware, 1992; Ware, 1984).

5. Face-to-face interaction time is the clinician's estimate of how much time was spent "face-to-face with this patient" during the screening visit, from less than five minutes to sixty minutes. Satisfaction with the visit is based on patients' responses to nine items rated on a five-point scale from poor to excellent. Items included the following: waiting time for an appointment, convenience of office location, ability to reach the office by telephone,

waiting time at the office, time spent with the provider, explanation of care provided, technical skills of the provider, personal manner of the provider, and the visit overall.

6. These percentages are predicted using the parameters of multiple regression models (logistic except for satisfaction with care, which is based on least-squares regression) and adjusted for all covariates (provider specialty, provider and patient demographics, and payment type). All models were adjusted for patient clustering within provider.

7. The COD obtained much more detail on the timing of episodes and remission than we used in analytic variables. Comparing reports of symptoms one year prior to the COD with contemporaneous reports of psychological distress from the relevant patient assessment questionnaires, we found that patients tended to compress the timing of the retrospective reports to be more consistent with their status at the time of the follow-up COD interview. Because of this bias, we were more confident of the occurrence of disorder and symptoms during the entire follow-up interval and during the last (most recent) month of the interval than we were of reports of exact timing of remote events during the prior year.

8. We included an observer measure of depressive symptoms that is perhaps the most commonly used outcome measure in depression clinical trials, the Hamilton Depression Rating Scale (Hamilton, 1967), in a structured version (Potts et al., 1990) for a subset of depressed patients.

9. These outcome measures required a lay-person telephone interviewer, but the computer-assisted administration greatly reduced training time, compared with the traditional DIS training, as well as errors in data collection, for example, those due to skip patterns in the diagnostic algorithm.

10. See McHorney et al., 1992, for a more detailed comparison of the validity and relative precision of MOS short- and long-form health status scales. The response rates for the depressed sample used for the psychometric analyses in this book varied on different instruments and at different phases of follow-up, but we weight the data for probability of response so that all the analyses refer to the baseline population.

11. Missing data at the item level for HRQOL scales are rare, and data completeness tends to be slightly lower for patients of general medical clinicians. Scale scoring rules, however, base the scores on nonmissing responses when some items have missing data, minimizing this problem.

12. Related to internal consistency is the issue of whether each item belongs in the scale to which it was assigned. The measure of item-total correlation indicates the range of correlations for each item with the set of others in a scale. Items should have an item-total correlation of at least 0.4, and with few exceptions, all items in our scales meet this standard. The exceptions are low item-total correlations for some items in the symptom

measure and general health perceptions. This is not unexpected considering their content, which was heterogeneous by design.

13. The pattern of these relationships is similar at baseline, year one, and year two.

14. For subthreshold patients, we observed an interesting pattern of associations with socially desirable responding: correlations of +0.22 for mental health (.22) but –0.22 for physical health, suggesting that patients may underreport psychological distress but overreport physical limitations due to socially desirable responding. That is, a somatic presentation of depression is more socially acceptable for this group.

6. Social and Clinical Factors

1. The correction is based on data from an independent study (Burnam et al., 1988). The prevalence findings are based on Burnam et al. (1995). Percentages across systems of care and specialty sectors are adjusted for differences in patient demographic factors and study site.

2. In analyses including form of organization (HMO, SOLO, MSG) rather than type of payment, there was a significant three-way interaction between site, system of care, and specialty, suggesting regional variations in whether HMOs or SOLO practices have a higher prevalence of patients with depression.

3. These results were first reported in Wells, Hays, et al. (1989).

4. The analysis used the more extensive measures of functioning and well-being that were collected in the smaller longitudinal panel. The constructs in the longitudinal study were the eight domains of the SF-36 described in Chapter 5. The scales had more items and higher reliability than the scales used for the cross-sectional analysis, however. The results are based on the full longitudinal sample of 1,790 depressed and nondepressed patients with complete data on baseline and two-year functioning and well-being. Type of depression or general medical conditions were the main independent variables in the linear regression models, and the covariates were age, education, income, gender, ethnicity, site, specialty, and type of payment at baseline.

5. Hypertensive patients were the only chronic condition group of sufficient size in the MOS to permit comparisons of depressed and nondepressed patients. All comparisons of family history and sickness were adjusted for patient demographic characteristics, study site, payment, and specialty using multiple (logistic and least-squares) regression models. See Sherbourne et al. (1994).

6. Provider choice was first analyzed in Sturm, Meredith, and Wells (forthcoming). We assigned treatment sector based on patient report of whether

or not the participating MOS clinician was the regular source of care, not necessarily limited to mental health problems only.

7. A simple way of estimating provider choice is through a qualitative response model, such as the multinomial logit model. Frank and Kamlet (1990) used this model to analyze choice of provider for persons with mental illness. This approach was not applicable for the MOS because patients were sampled according to their choice of provider, which is also known as endogenous or choice-based sampling. Instead, a choice-based sampling multinomial logit estimator was used (Amemiya, 1985). Choice-based sampling, which oversamples rare "choices," such as mental health specialists, increases the power to estimate the effect of health on provider specialty and is an advantage of the MOS. The disadvantage is that the choice-based estimation method requires precise knowledge of the ratio of the proportion of patients in a specialty sector in the study to the proportion of patients treated in the specialty sector. Because the dependent variable is the type of provider, we chose the weight corresponding to the sampling probability of the provider and controlled for other factors affecting the probability of patient selection by the regressor variables. See Sturm, Meredith, and Wells (forthcoming).

8. When we calculated the elasticities, the coefficients for psychological health implied that a 1 percent deterioration increased the probability of receiving care from a psychiatrist by about 1.1 percent and the probability of care from a nonphysician specialist by about 0.4 percent. When the analysis was restricted to the patients who considered this provider their regular source for mental health care, the effect was even stronger: a 1 percent deterioration in psychological health increased the probability of psychiatry care by 2.8 percent and the probability of other mental health specialty care by 1.1 percent. See Sturm, Meredith, and Wells (forthcoming).

9. This analysis used data on all 715 patients who completed the second-stage telephone DIS and had a current major depression or dysthymia, including two individuals not eligible for the longitudinal analysis. A number of measures are available only on a subset of these patients, however. The full results are given in Wells, Burnam, Rogers, and Camp (1995). The findings are adjusted for differences in patient demographic characteristics, but findings were similar with and without such adjustment. The covariates are age, gender, ethnicity, education, income, marital status, and site.

10. We also had a wider range of health status measures, but this is not the cause for the more recent findings of specialty differences (similar specialty differences seem to exist in the National Comorbidity Study [Frank, personal communication]). For example, Cooper-Patrick, Crum, and Ford (1994) relied primarily on indicators of lifetime symptom counts, whereas our analysis relied primarily on recent severity measures, but lifetime depressive symptoms also differed by specialty in our sample.

11. For patients with depressive symptoms but no lifetime depressive disorder, the depressive symptoms could likely reflect primary symptoms of a "comorbid" psychiatric illness. Focusing on patients with lifetime depressive disorder makes comorbid conditions more interpretable. Results are based on multiple logistic regression models. Covariates are gender, age, employment, marital status, ethnicity, study site, and presence or absence of current depressive disorder versus past depressive disorder. The full results are reported in Wells et al. (1991).

12. In an analysis of patients with current depressive disorder, Wells, Burnam, Rogers, and Camp (1995) examined specialty differences in a global measure of physical sickness, combining counts of chronic medical conditions and measures of physical functioning and well-being. After controlling for confounding demographic factors (particularly age), there were no significant specialty differences or payment differences in global physical sickness.

13. As with medical comorbidity, we analyzed psychiatric comorbidity for the sample with lifetime depressive disorder and controlled for confounding patient demographic factors. Panic disorder results are presented in Wells, Burnam, Rogers, and Camp (1995); alcoholism results in Sherbourne et al. (1993).

14. As in the comorbidity analyses, the main analysis examined differences in morbidity for patients with *lifetime* depressive disorder. The analysis relied on a set of nested regression models, first controlling for confounding patient demographic factors alone and then for demographic factors, depression, and chronic medical conditions. The sociodemographic variables were age, education, gender, ethnicity, marital status, family income, and site; the second analysis added an indicator of depression severity (count of depressive symptoms); and the third analysis added a count of chronic medical conditions. This analysis used the full HRQOL measures and all related items in the MOS that were collected at the time of the fuller baseline assessment (PAQ) (Stewart et al., 1993). This hierarchical modeling approach determines both differences among patient groups in morbidity and whether or not any observed differences are due to confounding with severity of depression, or presence or absence of medical comorbidities.

15. Using global measures of physical and psychological sickness (described in Rogers et al., 1993) and patient demographics, we found that this qualitative pattern also holds for all depressed patients (including those with depressive symptoms only). There are two reasons payment differences are not significant, despite the different mix of specialties by payment and different levels of sickness by specialty. One reason is that pooling heterogeneous patient groups (from different specialty sectors) can lower the precision by increasing the variance, despite the simultaneous increase in sample size. The

second is that there are some compensating effects, for example, measures on which PP patients are slightly (but not significantly) sicker than FFS patients.

7. How Treatment Differs by Specialty and Payment

1. These analyses are based on 650 patients who completed the second-stage telephone interview and had current depressive symptoms. The full analyses are presented in Wells, Hays, et al. (1989).

2. This analysis is based on 634 patients with depressive symptoms, including current depressive disorder, who enrolled and completed a baseline interview about medication use. The psychotropic medications in the MOS include antidepressant medications—mono- and heterocyclic antidepressant medications, MAOIs, and new types of antidepressant medications. SSRIs were introduced in the United States in the mid-1980s and were not used at baseline in the MOS but were common at follow-up. The minor tranquilizers include all antianxiety and sedative / hypnotic agents, excluding antidepressant and antipsychotic medications. More details are reported in Wells et al. (1994). Findings from this paper are reported with permission of the American Psychiatric Association.

3. The numbers in Figure 7.5 are unadjusted, but we obtain similar conclusions when stratifying by severity or adjusting for patient demographics and general health perceptions. The qualitative results also hold when enlarging the definition of the focus of counseling to include any emotional or personal problem, not just depression.

4. Switches between payment systems were analyzed in Sturm et al. (1994) using the full longitudinal sample of depressed patients. The analysis, as well as analyses of utilization of mental health services, excluded patients becoming uninsured because such patients have very different demand for services than insured FFS patients, but the group was too small for an independent analysis. We used a two-state Markov model, in which the probability of switching plans each year was modeled by a logistic regression equation.

5. The utilization results are based on Sturm, Jackson, et al. (1995). The analysis of visits uses the standard two-part model (Duan et al., 1983). The first part is a logit equation for the probability of any outpatient mental health care. The second part regresses the natural logarithm of the number of mental health visits on explanatory variables to analyze the level of use for patients with one or more visits. The first equation separates users from nonusers and addresses the large number of zero use. The logarithmic transformation of the number of visits for users in the second regression equation alleviates the skewness displayed by the data. To study the effect of switching between payment types on utilization, we analyzed the residual—actual

number of mental health visits minus predicted number—based on the two-part model including the logistic regression for probability of any visit and the logarithmic regression for number of visits among those with one or more visits. This approach detects systematic selection effects beyond those related to observable differences in patient characteristics.

Switchers and stayers appeared to differ along some unobserved dimensions, which might indicate systematic preferences for specific treatment settings. In particular, after adjusting for observed patient characteristics and health status, patients switching out of PP had higher baseline use than predicted, whereas patients switching out of FFS had lower use than predicted. Thus there appeared to be some biased selection that was *not* related to health status. We give only descriptive statistics in this chapter. The conclusions regarding payment system are unaffected by adjustments for demographics or health status, and switching had only a minor effect on utilization findings. For a different analysis of the relationship between utilization and appropriate care, see Chapter 9.

6. To address provider continuity, we used nonparametric and parametric duration models to analyze the time until a patient reported that he / she no longer considered the initial MOS clinician to be a source of care, using the longitudinal sample of depressed patients. The analysis included unadjusted and adjusted models, controlling for effects of baseline patient demographic characteristics, payment system, and global physical and psychological sickness, with similar conclusions. See Sturm, Meredith, and Wells (forthcoming) for details.

8. Health Outcomes

1. The clinical outcomes analysis used data on the 747 patients who participated in the telephone follow-up outcome study, which included patients with either current depressive disorder or current depressive symptoms, no current disorder, but having either a past disorder or just missing criteria for a past disorder. We examined level of symptoms or occurrence of disorder in each follow-up interval, controlling for baseline type and level of depression, patient demographic characteristics, and medical comorbidity (Wells et al., 1992).

2. Clinical studies have used change in either diagnostic status or number or severity of depressive symptoms as the clinical outcome measure, chiefly utilizing instruments such as the Beck Depression Inventory (BDI) or the Hamilton Depression Rating Scale (HDRS). We used a conceptually similar but less standard approach, namely, the count of current symptoms of DSM-III depressive disorders (major depressive or dysthymic disorder, or melancholia), and counts of spells of depression.

3. The FFS-PP outcome comparison was first reported in Rogers et al. (1993).

4. Some of the outcome difference clearly is related to switching, as the difference between PP and FFS patients of psychiatrists in outcomes is much reduced when analyzing differences using type of payment at the end of two years (rather than at baseline) as the indicator of payment type.

5. When one combines heterogeneous groups, such as pooling across specialty sectors, the increase in the variance may overwhelm the increased sample size and reduce the statistical power to find differences. Put differently, a system could be consistently and significantly worse in every single sector, but if these sectors are heterogeneous, the difference may not be statistically significant when one pools across them. This means not that the systems are performing similarly overall or that the overall difference is not important, but that different analyses have different statistical power, and a pooled analysis does not necessarily have better statistical power than a stratified analysis.

6. The difference between PP and FFS was primarily due to IPAs, however, and the FFS versus IPA comparison was significant at $p < .001$. Rogers et al. (1993) also tested for site effects by including an interaction term between geographic site and type of payment. The findings indicated that the PP effect was significant in two sites but not the third.

9. Cost-Effective Care

1. This chapter is based on Sturm and Wells (1995), which is adapted with permission of the American Medical Association.

2. If two delivery systems differ in the probability that a patient receives an efficacious treatment, a direct outcomes comparison by delivery system may be unable to detect a difference with sample sizes of a few hundred because outcomes are highly variable due to the mix of treated and untreated cases. In contrast, an indirect analysis may have good power to detect a difference in probability of treatment by system and good power to detect the treatment-outcomes relationships with the same sample size. In fact, the high natural variability in many outcomes measures, combined with a high variability in treatment rates across patients, may make it extremely difficult to detect even moderately large outcomes differences between different health care systems unless there are extremely large samples, that is, much larger than the MOS. There is a risk that outcome measurement can be used to justify a lower level of quality of care.

3. The best process-of-care measures were available at baseline only. For example, we had no information about counseling or psychotherapy beyond the baseline visit, and it is not even clear how to model the link between

counseling and outcome over time because psychotherapy's efficacy is controversial in the continuation phase (Depression Guidelines Panel, 1993b). Kamlet et al. (1992) developed a first model to analyze the cost-effectiveness in the continuation therapy of a clinical trial, but the data and conceptual problems of the continuation and maintenance phases in actual practice settings, such as the role of plan switching, need to be addressed in future studies of treatment in usual care settings.

4. The cost for a psychiatry visit ($120) is a weighted average of continuing therapy and initial assessment costs, based on the American Medical Association's 1993 Physician Marketplace Statistics. The lower cost for a visit to a nonphysician mental health specialist ($100) reflects differences in training. We weighted a visit to a general medical clinician at $60, which reflects the visit cost for a *new* patient in general medical practices, rather than the cost for an established patient ($40) or a weighted average. Our reasoning was that appropriate care for these particular patients is more demanding than a typical visit of an established general medical patient. This assumption may overestimate the costs per patient under care as usual, but our qualitative conclusions are not affected even if improving quality of care raises not only utilization but also the costs for each visit in the general medical sector from $40 to $60. We weighted monthly pharmacy costs by the number of patients receiving each medication, using 1993 costs. We estimated the average costs for minor tranquilizers to be about $225 for six months and the average costs of antidepressants to be around $170 for nine months. With the development of new antidepressant medications, this relationship has changed, but the conclusions are not sensitive to large changes in medication costs (even a tripling) because they are a relatively small component of total costs.

5. We can analyze FFS care similarly, but we focus on PP managed care here because it reflects the national trend toward greater reliance on managed-care strategies and because we found greater need for quality improvement in PP care. The same principles also apply for analyzing care for less seriously ill patients, but there is one important caveat: we found no evidence that any processes of care were significantly associated with better or worse outcomes for less sick patients.

6. The Serious Limitations measure is the number of four serious limitations in daily role and physical functioning (not able to work at a paying job, not able to do housework, not able to do strenuous exercise such as lawn mowing, not able to do moderate exercise such as climbing stairs). We analyze change in limitations from baseline to the end of the second year of follow-up.

7. We estimated the probability that a patient receives a certain type of treatment using qualitative response regression models to adjust for confounding factors—in particular, initial sickness and patient demographics.

8. Note the absence of a detection node in Figure 9.1. If detection is the only process-of-care variable included in an outcomes analysis, its (significant) coefficient suggests that detection leads to larger improvements and better outcomes. But when medication and counseling are modeled, detection becomes insignificant and is only associated with a minor adverse effect on outcomes, which probably represents unmeasured sickness characteristics. Clearly, detection does not make patients worse off, and it therefore would be misleading to include this residual chronicity or sickness effect of detection in our model of the effects of processes of care. Such a model would have the absurd implication that the best treatment for patients is not to detect their depression, but to counsel them for depression and provide antidepressant medication. Of course, detection by itself does not make patients better either. What matters is appropriate treatment, not detection. The importance of detection stems from its focal point as a necessary step to instituting treatment, implying an important role in quality-improvement interventions, a large research area.

References

Abraham, Karl. 1948. *Selected Papers of Karl Abraham.* London: Hogarth Press.

Alchin, Terry M., and Henry W. Tranby. 1994. "Who Bears the Cost of Antidepressants in Australia?" *Medical Journal of Australia* 161(9):547–549.

Amemiya, Takeshi. 1985. *Advanced Econometrics.* Cambridge, Mass.: Harvard University Press.

American Psychiatric Association. 1993. "Practice Guideline for Major Depressive Disorder in Adults." *American Journal of Psychiatry* 150 (April suppl.):1029.

Attkisson, C. Clifford, and Jane M. Zich. 1990. *Depression in Primary Care: Screening and Detection.* New York: Routledge.

Bach, Stephen. 1994. "Managing a Pluralist Health System: The Case of Health Care Reform in France." *International Journal of Health Services* 24(4):593–606.

Bachrach, Leona L. 1993. "Continuity of Care and Approaches to Case Management for Long-Term Mentally Ill Patients." *Hospital and Community Psychiatry* 44(5):465–468.

Badger, Lee W., and Elizabeth H. Rand. 1988. "Unlearning Psychiatry: A Cohort Effect in the Training Environment." *International Journal of Psychiatry in Medicine* 18:123–135.

Beck, Aaron T. 1962. "Thinking and Depression II: Theory and Therapy." *Archives of General Psychiatry* 10:561–571.

——— 1967a. *Cognitive Therapy and the Emotional Disorders.* New York: International Universities Press, Inc., pp. 116–119.

——— 1967b. *Depression: Clinical, Experimental, and Theoretical Aspects.* New York: Harper and Row.

Berry, Sandra H. 1992. "Methods of Collecting Health Data." In Anita L. Stewart and John E. Ware, Jr., eds., *Measuring Functioning and Well-*

Being: The Medical Outcomes Study Approach. Durham, N.C.: Duke University Press, pp. 48–66.

Billings, Andrew G., Ruth C. Cronkite, and Rudolf H. Moos. 1983. "Social-Environmental Factors in Unipolar Depression: Comparisons of Depressed Patients and Nondepressed Controls." *Journal of Abnormal Psychology* 92(2):119–133.

Billings, Andrew G., and Rudolf H. Moos. 1984. "Treatment Experiences of Adults with Unipolar Depression: The Influence of Patient and Life Context Factors." *Journal of Consulting and Clinical Psychology* 92:119–133.

Blanchard, M. R., A. Waterreus, and A. H. Mann. 1994. "The Nature of Depression among Older People in Inner London, and the Contact with Primary Care." *British Journal of Psychiatry* 164(396):396–402.

Blazer, Dan G., Ronald C. Kessler, Katherine A. McGonagle, and Marvin S. Swartz. 1994. "The Prevalence and Distribution of Major Depression in a National Community Sample: The National Comorbidity Study." *American Journal of Psychiatry* 151(7):979–986.

Bound, John, David A. Jaeger, and Regina M. Baker. 1995. "Problems with Instrumental Variables Estimation When the Correlation between the Instruments and the Endogenous Explanatory Variable Is Weak." *Journal of the American Statistical Association* 90(430):443.

Brazier, J. E., R. Harper, N. M. B. Jones, A. O'Caithain, K. J. Thomas, T. Usherwood, and L. Westlake. 1992. "Validating the SF-36 Health Survey Questionnaire: New Outcome Measure for Primary Care." *British Medical Journal* 305:160–164.

Broadhead, Jeremy, and Melanie Abas. 1994. "Depressive Illness—Zimbabwe." *Tropical Doctor* 24(1):27–30.

Broadhead, W. Eugene, Dan G. Blazer, Linda K. George, and Chiu Kit Tse. 1990. "Depression, Disability Days, and Days Lost from Work in a Prospective Epidemiologic Survey." *Journal of the American Medical Association* 264(19):2524–2528.

Brody, David S., Caryn E. Lerman, Heidi Wolfson, and G. Craig Caputo. 1990. "Improvement in Physicians' Counseling of Patients with Mental Health Problems." *Archives of Internal Medicine* 150:993–998.

Bromet, Evelyn J., David K. Parkinson, Carroll Curtis, Herbert C. Schulberg, Howard Blane, Leslie O. Dunn, Jo Phelan, Mary A. Dew, and Joseph E. Schwartz. 1990. "Epidemiology of Depression and Alcohol Abuse / Dependence in a Managerial and Professional Work Force." *Journal of Occupational Medicine* 32(10):989–995.

Brown, Diane R., Feroz Ahmed, Lawrence E. Gary, and Norweeta G. Milburn. 1995. "Major Depression in a Community Sample of African Americans." *American Journal of Psychiatry* 152(3):373–378.

Bryk, Anthony S., and Stephen W. Raudenbush. 1992. *Hierarchical Linear Models: Applications and Data Analysis Methods.* Newbury Park, Calif.: Sage Publications.

Burnam, M. Audrey, Kenneth B. Wells, Barbara Leake, and John Lansverk. 1988. "Development of a Brief Screening Instrument for Detecting Depressive Disorders." *Medical Care* 26(8):775–789.

Burnam, M. Audrey, Kenneth B. Wells, William Rogers, Marilyn K. Potts, and John Ware, Jr. 1995. *Prevalence of Depression in General Medical and Mental Health Outpatient Practices in Three Health Care Systems.* Publication no. P-7956. Santa Monica, Calif.: RAND.

Caldecott-Hazard, Sally, Barry H. Guze, Mitchel A. Kling, Arthur Kling, and Lewis R. Baxter. 1991. "Clinical and Biochemical Aspects of Depressive Disorders: I. Introduction, Classification, and Research Techniques." *Synapse* 8:185–211.

Caldecott-Hazard, Sally, David G. Morgan, Frank DeLeon-Jones, David H. Overstreet, and David Janowsky. 1991. "Clinical and Biochemical Aspects of Depressive Disorders: II. Transmitter / Receptor Theories." *Synapse* 9:251–301.

Caldecott-Hazard, Sally, and Lon S. Schneider. 1992. "Clinical and Biochemical Aspects of Depressive Disorders: III. Treatment and Controversies." *Synapse* 10(2):141–168.

Campbell, Donald T. 1957. "Factors Relevant to the Validity of Experiments in Social Settings." *Psychological Bulletin* 54:297–312.

Chamberlain, Gary. 1984. Panel Data. *Handbook of Econometrics.* Amsterdam: North Holland.

Cook, Thomas D., and Donald T. Campbell. 1979. *Quasi-Experimentation: Design and Analysis Issues for Field Settings.* Chicago: Rand McNally.

Cook, Thomas D., and William R. Shadish. 1994. "Social Experiments: Some Developments over the Past Fifteen Years." *Annual Review of Psychology* 45:545–580.

Cooper-Patrick, Lisa, Rosa M. Crum, and Daniel E. Ford. 1994. "Characteristics of Patients with Major Depression Who Received Care in General Medical and Specialty Mental Health Settings." *Medical Care* 32:15–24.

Coryell, William, Jean Endicott, and Martin Keller. 1990. "Outcome of Patients with Chronic Affective Disorder: A Five-Year Follow-Up." *American Journal of Psychiatry* 147:1627–1633.

Coulehan, John L., Herbert C. Schulberg, Marian R. Block, and Monica Zettler-Segal. 1988. "Symptom Patterns of Depression in Ambulatory Medical and Psychiatric Patients." *Journal of Nervous and Mental Disease* 176:284–288.

Coulehan, John L., Herbert C. Schulberg, Marian R. Block, et al. 1990.

"Medical Comorbidity of Major Depressive Disorder in a Primary Medical Practice." *Archives of Internal Medicine* 150:2363–2367.

Covi, Lino, and Ronald S. Lipman. 1987. "Cognitive Behavioral Group Psychotherapy Combined with Imipramine in Major Depression." *Psychopharmacological Bulletin* 23:173–176.

Cronbach, Lee J. 1951. "Coefficient Alpha and the Internal Structure of Tests." *Psychometrika* 16:297–334.

Cross-National Collaborative Group. 1992. "The Changing Rate of Major Depression: Cross-National Comparisons." *Journal of the American Medical Association* 268(21):3098–3105.

Depression Guidelines Panel. 1993a. *Depression in Primary Care: Volume 1. Detection and Diagnosis.* U.S. Department of Health and Human Services, Public Health Service, Agency for Health Care Policy and Research, AHCPR Publication no. 93–0550. Rockville, Md.: AHCPR.

——— 1993b. *Depression in Primary Care: Volume 2. Treatment of Major Depression.* U.S. Department of Health and Human Services, Public Health Service, Agency for Health Care Policy and Research, AHCPR Publication no. 93–0551. Rockville, Md.: AHCPR.

Diehr, Paula, Kurt Price, Stephen J. Williams, and Diane P. Martin. 1985. "Use of Outpatients Somatic Health Services by Patients Who Use or Need Mental Health Services in Three Provider Plans." *Journal of Medical Systems* 9:389–400.

Diehr, Paula, Stephen J. Williams, Diane P. Martin, and Kurt Price. 1984. "Ambulatory Mental Health Services Utilization in Three Provider Plans." *Medical Care* 22:1–13.

Donabedian, Avis. 1988. "The Quality of Care: How Can It Be Assessed?" *Journal of the American Medical Association* 260:1743–1748.

Donald, Cathy, and John E. Ware, Jr. 1982. *The Quantification of Social Contacts and Resources.* Publication no. R-2937-HHS. Santa Monica, Calif.: RAND.

Drummond, Michael F., Greg L. Stoddard, and George W. Torrance. 1987. *Methods for the Economic Evaluation of Health Care Programmes.* New York: Oxford University Press.

Duan, Naihua, Willard G. Manning, Carl N. Morris, and Joseph P. Newhouse. 1983. "A Comparison of Alternative Models for the Demand of Medical Care." *Journal of Business and Economic Statistics* 1(2):115–126.

Eisenberg, John. 1989. "Clinical Economics: A Guide to the Economic Analysis of Clinical Practices." *Journal of the American Medical Association* 262(20):2879–2886.

Elkin, Irene, M. Tracie Shea, John T. Watkins, Stanley D. Imber, Stuart M. Sotsky, Joseph F. Collins, David R. Glass, Paul A. Pilkonis, William R. Leber, John P. Docherty, Susan J. Fiester, and Morris B. Parloff. 1989.

"National Institute of Mental Health Treatment of Depression Collaborative Research Program: General Effectiveness of Treatments." *Archives of General Psychiatry* 46(10):971–982.

Ellis, Randall P., and Thomas G. McGuire. 1993. "Supply-Side and Demand-Side Cost Sharing in Health Care." *Journal of Economic Perspectives* 7(4):135–151.

Ellwood, Paul. 1988. "Outcomes Management: A Technology of Patient Experience (Shattack Lecture)." *New England Journal of Medicine* 318(23):1549–1556.

Fenichel, Otto. 1945. "Depression and Mania." In *The Psychoanalytic Theory of Neurosis.* New York: W. W. Norton.

Fitzmaurice, Garrett M., Nan M. Laird, and Andrea G. Rotnitzky. 1993. "Regression Models for Discrete Longitudinal Responses." *Statistical Science* 8:284–309.

Ford, Daniel E. 1994. "Recognition and Underrecognition of Mental Disorders in Adult Primary Care." In Jeanne Miranda, Ann A. Hohmann, C. Clifford Attkisson, and David B. Larson, eds., *Mental Disorders in Primary Care.* San Francisco, Calif.: Jossey-Bass Publishers, Inc., pp. 186–205.

Frank, Ellen, David J. Kupfer, Cleon Cornes, and Susan M. Morris. 1993. "Maintenance Interpersonal Psychotherapy for Recurrent Depression." In Gerald L. Klerman and Myrna M. Weissman, eds., *New Applications of Interpersonal Psychotherapy.* Washington, D.C.: American Psychiatric Press, Inc., pp. 75–102.

Frank, Ellen, David J. Kupfer, J. M. Perel, Cleon Cornes, D. B. Jarrett, A. G. Mallinger, M. E. Thase, Ann B. McEachran, and V. J. Grochocinski. 1990. "Three-Year Outcomes for Maintenance Therapies in Recurrent Depression." *Archives of General Psychiatry* 47:1093–1099.

Frank, Ellen, David J. Kupfer, Eric F. Wagner, Ann B. McEachran, and Cleon Cornes. 1991. "Efficacy of Interpersonal Psychotherapy as a Maintenance Treatment of Recurrent Depression: Contributing Factors." *Archives of General Psychiatry* 48:1053–1059.

Frank, Jerome D. 1961. *Persuasion and Healing: A Comparative Study of Psychotherapy.* Baltimore, Md.: Johns Hopkins University Press.

Frank, Richard G., and Paul J. Gertler. 1991. "An Assessment of Measurement Error Bias for Estimating the Effect of Mental Distress on Income." *Journal of Human Resources* 26(1):154–164.

Frank, Richard G., and Mark S. Kamlet. 1989. "Determining Provider Choice for the Treatment of Mental Disorder: The Role of Health and Mental Status." *Health Services Research* 24:83–103.

——— 1990. "Economic Aspects of Patterns of Mental Health Care: Cost Variation by Setting." *General Hospital Psychiatry* 12(1):11–18.

Frank, Richard G., and Thomas J. McGuire. 1986. "A Review of Studies of the Impact of Insurance on the Demand and Utilization of Specialty Mental Health Services." *Health Services Research* 21 (Part II):241–265.

Freud, Sigmund. 1917. *Mourning and Melancholia.* Standard Edition, Volume 14 (1955). London: Hogarth Press, pp. 737–858.

Geigle, Ron, and Stanley B. Jones. 1990. "Outcomes Measurement: A Report from the Front." *Inquiry* 27:7–13.

George, Linda K., Dan G. Blazer, Dana G. Hughes, and Nancy Fowler. 1989. "Social Support and the Outcome of Major Depression." *British Journal of Psychiatry* 154:478–485.

Gerber, Paul D., James Barrett, Jane Barrett, Eric Manheimer, Richard Whiting, and Robert Smith. 1989. "Recognition of Depression in Internists in Primary Care: A Comparison of Internist and Gold Standard Psychiatric Assessments." *Journal of General Internal Medicine* 4:7–13.

German, Pearl S., Sam Shapiro, Elizabeth A. Skinner, Michael Von Korgg, Lawrence E. Klein, Raymond W. Turner, Mark L. Teitelbaum, Jack Burke, and Barbara J. Burns. 1987. "Detection and Management of Mental Health Problems of Older Patients by Primary Care Providers." *Journal of the American Medical Association* 257(4):489–493.

Gershon, Eliot S., Wade H. Berrettini, John I. Nurnberger, Jr., and Lynn R. Goldin. 1989. "Genetic Studies of Affective Illness." In J. John Mann, M.D., ed., *Models of Depressive Disorders.* New York: Plenum Press.

Gertler, Paul, and Roland Sturm. Forthcoming. "Using Private Health Insurance to Reduce and Better Target Public Expenditures." *Journal of Econometrics.*

Gibbons, Robert D., Donald Hedeker, Irene Elkin, Christine Waternaux, Helena C. Kraemer, Joel B. Greenhouse, M. Tracie Shea, Stanley D. Imber, Stuart M. Sotsky, and John T. Watkins. 1993. "Some Conceptual and Statistical Issues in Analysis of Longitudinal Psychiatric Data." *Archives of General Psychiatry* 50(9):739–750.

Giles, Donna E., David Kupfer, Howard Roffwarg, A. John Rush, Melanie M. Biggs, and Barbara A. Etzel. 1989. "Polysomnographic Parameters in First-Degree Relatives of Unipolar Probands." *Psychiatry Research* 27(2):127–136.

Gitlin, Michael. 1990. *The Psychotherapist's Guide to Psychopharmacology.* New York: The Free Press, pp. 17–78.

Goldberg, David, and Y. Lecrubier. 1995. "Form and Frequency of Mental Disorders across Centres." In T. B. Üstün and N. Sartorius, *Mental Illness in General Health Care: An International Study.* New York: John Wiley and Sons, pp. 323–334.

Goldberg, David, Jane J. Steele, Alan Johnson, and Charles Smith. 1982.

"Ability of Primary Care Physicians to Make Accurate Ratings of Psychiatric Symptoms." *Archives of General Psychiatry* 39(7):829–833.

Greenberg, Paul E., Laura E. Stiglin, Stan N. Finkelstein, and Ernst R. Berndt. 1993. "The Economic Burden of Depression in 1990." *Journal of Clinical Psychiatry* 54:405–418.

Greenhouse, J. B., D. Stangl, D. J. Kupfer, and R. F. Prien. 1991. "Methodologic Issues in Maintenance Therapy Clinical Trials." *Archives of General Psychiatry* 48:313–318.

Greenley, James R., David Mechanic, and Paul D. Cleary. 1987. "Seeking Help for Psychologic Problems: A Replication and Extension." *Medical Care* 25(12):1113–1128.

Grove, William M., and Nancy C. Andreasen. 1992. "Concepts, Diagnosis, and Classification." In Eugene S. Paykel, ed., *Handbook of Affective Disorders*. New York: The Guilford Press, pp. 25–41.

Haas, Gretchen L., and Marion L. Fitzgibbon. 1989. "Cognitive Models." In John J. Mann, ed., *Models of Depressive Disorders—Psychological, Biological, and Genetic Perspectives*. The Depressive Illness Series, Volume 2. New York: Plenum Press, pp. 9–43.

Hamilton, Max. 1967. "Development of a Rating Scale for Primary Depressive Illness." *British Journal of Social and Clinical Psychology* 6(4):278–296.

Hankin, Janet R., and Ben Z. Locke. 1982. "The Persistence of Depressive Symptomatology among Prepaid Group Practice Enrollees: An Exploratory Study." *American Journal of Public Health* 72(9):1000–1007.

Hankin, Janet R., and Julianne S. Oktay. 1979. *Mental Disorder and Primary Medical Care: An Analytical Review of Literature*. NIMH, series D, no. 5, DHEW Publication no. (ADM) 78–661. Washington, D.C.: U.S. Government Printing Office.

Hays, Ronald D., Cathy D. Sherbourne, and Rebecca Mazel. 1993. "The RAND 36-Item Health Survey 1.0." *Health Economics* 2(3):217–227.

Hays, Ronald D., and Anita L. Stewart. 1990. "The Structure of Self-Reported Health in Chronic Disease Patients." *Psychiatric Assessment* 2:22–30.

Hays, Ronald D., Kenneth B. Wells, Cathy D. Sherbourne, William Rogers, and Karen Spritzer. 1995. "Functioning and Well-Being Outcomes of Patients with Depression Compared with Chronic General Medical Illnesses." *Archives of General Psychiatry* 52(1):11–19.

Heckman, James J. 1990. "Varieties of Selection Bias." *American Economic Review* 80:313–318.

Heckman, James J., and V. Joseph Hotz. 1989. "Choosing among Alternative Nonexperimental Methods for Estimating the Impact of Social Programs: The Case of Manpower Training." *Journal of the American Statistical Association* 84:862–874.

Heckman, James J., and Jeffrey A. Smith. 1995. "Assessing the Case for Social Experiments." *Journal of Economic Perspectives* 9:85–110.

Helmstadter, G. C. 1964. *Principles of Psychological Measurement.* New York: Appleton Century Crofts.

Helzer, John E., Lee N. Robins, Larry T. McEvoy, Edward L. Spitznagel, Roger K. Stoltzman, Anne Farmer, and Ian F. Brockington. 1985. "A Comparison of Clinical and Diagnostic Interview Schedule Diagnoses: Physician Reexamination of Lay-Interviewed Cases in the General Population." *Archives of General Psychiatry* 42(7):657–666.

Hennessey, John C., and Janice M. Dykacs. 1989. "Projected Outcomes and Length of Time in the Disability Insurance Program." *Social Security Bulletin* 52(9):2–41.

Hoeper, Edwin W., Gregory R. Nycz, Larry G. Kessler, Jack D. Burke, Jr., and Willard E. Pierce. 1984. "The Usefulness of Screening for Mental Illness." *The Lancet* 1:33–35.

Holsboer, Florian. 1995. "Neuroendocrinology of Mood Disorders." In Floyd Bloom and David Kupfer, eds., *Psychopharmacology: The Fourth Generation of Progress.* New York: Raven Press, pp. 957–970.

Hoy, Elizabeth W., R. E. Curtis, and Tom Rice. 1991. "Change and Growth in Managed Care." *Health Affairs* 10(4):18–35.

Hsiao, Cheng. 1986. *Analysis of Panel Data.* Econometric Society Monographs no. 11. New York: Cambridge University Press.

Huber, Peter J. 1967. *The Behavior of Maximum Likelihood Estimates under Nonstandard Conditions.* Fifth Berkeley Symposium on Mathematical Statistics and Probability 1:221–233.

Huff, D. 1954. *How to Lie with Statistics.* New York: W. W. Norton.

Huszonek, John J., Mantosh J. Dewan, Marvin Koss, William J. Hardoby, and Abbas Ispahani. 1993. "Antidepressant Side Effects and Physician Prescribing Patterns." *Annals of Clinical Psychiatry* 5(1):7–11.

Jacobsen, E. 1941. *Depression: Comparative Studies of Normal, Neurotic, and Psychotic Conditions.* New York: International Universities Press.

Jenkinson, Crispin, Angeles Coulter, and Lucie Wright. 1993. "Short Form 36 (SF 36) Health Survey Questionnaire: Normative Data for Adults of Working Age." *British Medical Journal* 306(6890):1437–1440.

Johnson, D. A .W. 1973. "Treatment of Depression in General Practice." *British Medical Journal* 2(5857):18–20.

Johnson, Jim, Myrna M. Weissman, and Gerald L. Klerman. 1992. "Service Utilization and Social Morbidity Associated with Depressive Symptoms in the Community." *Journal of the American Medical Association* 267(11):1478–1483.

Kamlet, Mark S. 1992. *The Comparative Benefit Modeling Project: A Frame-*

work for Cost-Utility Analysis of Government Health Care Programs. Bethesda, Md.: Report to the Office of Disease Prevention and Health Promotion. Public Health Service, U.S. Department of Health and Human Services.

Kamlet, Mark S., Mitchell Wade, David J. Kupfer, and Ellen Frank. 1992. "Cost-Utility Analysis of Maintenance Treatment for Recurrent Depression: A Theoretical Framework and Numerical Illustration." In Richard G. Frank and W. G. Manning, Jr., eds., *Economics and Mental Health.* Baltimore, Md.: Johns Hopkins University Press.

Kaplan, Robert M., and John P. Anderson. 1988. "A General Health Policy Model: Update and Applications." *Health Services Research* 23(2):203–235.

Kaplan, Robert M., J. W. Bush, and C. C. Berry. 1976. "Health Status: Types of Validity for an Index of Well-Being." *Health Services Research* 11:478–507.

Kaplan, Sherrie H., Sheldon Greenfield, and John E. Ware, Jr. 1989. "Assessing the Effects of Physician-Patient Interactions on the Outcome of Chronic Disease." *Medical Care* 27(3):S110–S127.

Katon, Wayne, and Herbert C. Schulberg. 1992. "Epidemiology of Depression in Primary Care." *General Hospital Psychiatry* 14(4):237–247.

Katon, Wayne, and Mark D. Sullivan. 1990. "Depression and Chronic Medical Illness." *Journal of Clinical Psychiatry* 51(Suppl):3–14.

Katon, Wayne, Michael Von Korff, Elizabeth Lin, T. Bush, and Johann Ormel. 1992. "Adequacy of Duration of Antidepressant Treatment in Primary Care." *Medical Care* 30:67–76.

Katon, Wayne, Michael Von Korff, Elizabeth Lin, Edward Walker, Greg E. Simon, Terry Bush, Patricia Robinson, and Joan Russo. 1995. "Collaborative Management to Achieve Treatment Guidelines: Impact on Depression in Primary Care." *Journal of the American Medical Association* 273(13):1026–1031.

Keeler, Emmett B., Willard G. Manning, and Kenneth B. Wells. 1988. "The Demand for Episodes of Mental Health Services." *Journal of Health Economics* 7:369–392.

Keller, Martin B., Philip W. Lavori, Jean Endicott, William Coryell, and Gerald L. Klerman. 1983. "Double Depression: Two-Year Follow-Up." *American Journal of Psychiatry* 140(6):689–694.

Keller, Martin B., Philip W. Lavori, Gerald L. Klerman, Nancy C. Andreasen, Jean Endicott, William Coryell, Jan Fawcett, John P. Rice, and M. A. Robert. 1986. "Low Levels and Lack of Predictors of Somatotherapy and Psychotherapy Received by Depressed Patients." *Archives of General Psychiatry* 43(5):458–466.

Keller, Martin B., Philip W. Lavori, Collins E. Lewis, and Gerald L. Klerman. 1983. "Predictors of Relapse in Major Depressive Disorder." *Journal of the American Medical Association* 250(24):3299–3304.

Keller, Martin B., Robert W. Shapiro, Philip W. Lavori, and Nicola Wolfe. 1982. "Relapse in Major Depressive Disorder—Analysis with the Life Table." *Archives of General Psychiatry* 39(8):911–915.

Kelly, Kevin, and Arnold M. Cooper. 1989. "Intrapsychic Models." In John J. Mann, ed., *Models of Depressive Disorders: Psychological, Biological, and Genetic Perspectives.* New York: Plenum Press, pp. 79–91.

Kendler, Kenneth, Ronald C. Kessler, Ellen E. Walters, Charles Maclean, Michael Neale, Andrew C. Heath, and Lindon J. Eaves. 1995. "Stressful Life Events, Genetic Liability, and Onset of an Episode of Major Depression in Women." *American Journal of Psychiatry* 152(6):833–842.

Kessler, Larry G., Donald M. Steinwachs, and Janet R. Hankin. 1980. "Episodes of Psychiatric Utilization." *Medical Care* 8:1219–1227.

Kessler, Larry G., Benjamin C. Amick II, and James Thompson. 1985. "Factors Influencing the Diagnosis of Mental Disorder among Primary Care Patients." *Medical Care* 23(1):50–62.

Kessler, Larry G., Paul D. Cleary, and Jack D. Burke, Jr. 1985. "Psychiatric Disorders in Primary Care: Results of a Follow-Up Study." *Archives of General Psychiatry* 42(6):583–587.

Kessler, Ronald C., Katherine A. McGonagle, Shanyang Zhao, Christopher B. Nelson, Michael Hughes, Suzann Eshlerman, Hans-Ulrich Wittchen, Kenneth S. Kendler. 1994. "Lifetime and Twelve-Month Prevalence of DSM-III-R Psychiatric Disorders in the United States: Results from the National Comorbidity Survey." *Archives of General Psychiatry* 51(1):8–19.

Kessner, David M., Carolyn E. Kalk, and James Singer. 1973. "Assessing Health Quality—The Case for Tracers." *New England Journal of Medicine* 288(4):189–194.

Kind, P., and J. Sorensen. 1993. "The Costs of Depression." *International Clinical Psychopharmacology* 7(3–4):191–195.

Kivela, Sirkka-Liisa, and Kimmo Pahkala. 1989. "Dysthymic Disorder in the Aged in the Community." *Social Psychiatry and Psychiatric Epidemiology* 24(2):77–83.

Klein, Daniel N., Ellen B. Taylor, Kathryn Harding, and Susan Dickstein. 1988. "Double Depression and Episodic Major Depression: Demographic, Clinical, Familial, Personality, and Socioenvironmental Characteristics and Short-Term Outcome." *American Journal of Psychiatry* 145(10):1226–1231.

Klein, Melanie. 1948. "A Contribution to the Psychogenesis of the Manic-Depressive States: Mourning and Its Relation to Manic-Depressive

States." In *Contributions to Psychoanalysis, 1921–1945*. London: Hogarth, pp. 282–338.

Klerman, Gerald L. 1980. "Other Specific Affective Disorders." In Harold I. Kaplan, Alfred M. Freedman, and Benjamin J. Sadock, eds., *Comprehensive Textbook of Psychiatry / III, Volume 2*. Baltimore, Md.: Williams and Wilkins.

———— 1987. "Clinical Epidemiology of Suicide." *Journal of Clinical Psychiatry* 48(12)(Suppl):33–38.

———— 1989a. "The Interpersonal Model." In John J. Mann, ed., *Models of Depressive Disorders: Psychological, Biological, and Genetic Perspectives*. New York: Plenum Press, pp. 45–77.

———— 1989b. "Psychiatric Diagnostic Categories: Issues of Validity and Measurement—An Invited Comment on Mirowsky and Ross (1989)." *Journal of Health and Social Behavior* 30(1):26–32.

Klerman, Gerald L., and Myrna M. Weissman. 1989. "Increasing Rates of Depression." *Journal of the American Medical Association* 261:2229–2235.

———— 1993. *New Applications of Interpersonal Psychotherapy*. Washington, D.C.: American Psychiatric Press, Inc.

Kupfer, David J. 1991. "Long-Term Treatment of Depression." *Journal of Clinical Psychiatry* 52(Suppl):28–34.

Kupfer, David J., and Charles F. Reynolds. 1992. "Sleep and Affective Disorders." In Eugene S. Paykel, ed., *Handbook of Affective Disorders*. New York: The Guilford Press, pp. 311–323.

LaLonde, Robert. 1986. "Evaluating the Econometric Evaluations of Training Programs with Experimental Data." *American Economic Review* 76(4):604–620.

Leaf, Philip J., Martha Livingston Bruce, and Gary L. Tischler. 1986. "The Differential Effects of Attitudes on the Use of Mental Health Services." *Social Psychiatry* 21(4):187–192.

Leaf, Philip J., Martha Livingston Bruce, Gary L. Tischler, Daniel H. Freeman, Jr., Myrna M. Weissman, and Jerome K. Myers. 1988. "Factors Affecting the Utilization of Specialty and General Medical Mental Health Services." *Medical Care* 26(1):9–26.

Leaf, Philip J., Martha M. Livingston, Gary L. Tischler, Myrna M. Weissman, Charles E. Holzer III, and Jerome K. Myers. 1985. "Contact with Health Professionals for the Treatment of Psychiatric and Emotional Problems." *Medical Care* 23:1322–1337.

Leamer, Edward E. 1983. "Let's Take the Con out of Econometrics." *American Economic Review* 73:31–43.

———— 1985. "Sensitivity Analyses Would Help." *American Economic Review* 75:308–313.

Lehtinen, V., and M. Joukamaa. 1994. "Epidemiology of Depression: Prevalence, Risk Factors, and Treatment Situation." *Acta Psychiatrica Scandinavia.* Suppl 377:7–10.

Lemelin, Jacques, Steve Hotz, Robert Swensen, and Thomas Elmslie. 1994. "Depression in Primary Care: Why Do We Miss the Diagnosis?" *Canadian Family Physician* 40(104):104–108.

Liang, Kung-Yee, and Scott L. Zeger. 1986. "Longitudinal Data Analysis Using Generalized Linear Models." *Biometrika* 73(1):13–22.

Linn, Lawrence S., and Joel S. Yager. 1982. "Screening of Depression in Relationship to Subsequent Patient and Physician Behavior." *Medical Care* 20(11):1233–1240.

Lurie, Nicole, Ira S. Moscovice, Michael Finch, Jon B. Christianson, and Michael K. Popkin. 1992. "Does Capitation Affect the Health of the Chronically Mentally Ill? Results from a Randomized Trial." *Journal of the American Medical Association* 267(24):3300–3304.

Madianos, M. G., and C. N. Stefanis. 1992. "Changes in the Prevalence of Symptoms of Depression and Depression across Greece." *Social Psychiatry and Psychiatric Epidemiology* 27:211–219.

Magruder-Habib, Kathryn, William K. Zung, and John R. Feussner. 1990. "Improving Physicians' Recognition and Treatment of Depression in General Medical Care: Results from a Randomized Clinical Trial." *Medical Care* 28(3):239–250.

Magruder-Habib, Kathryn, William K. Zung, John R. Feussner, Wendy C. Alling, William B. Saunders, and Holly Stevens. 1989. "Management of General Medical Patients with Symptoms of Depression." *General Hospital Psychiatry* 11(3):201–207.

Mann, John J., ed. 1989. *Models of Depressive Disorders: Psychological, Biological, and Genetic Perspectives.* New York: Plenum Press.

Manning, Willard G., Jr., Joseph P. Newhouse, and John E. Ware, Jr. 1982. "The Status of Health in Demand Estimation; or Beyond Excellent, Good, Fair, and Poor." In Victor R. Fuchs, ed., *Economic Aspects of Health.* Chicago, Ill.: National Bureau of Economic Research, University of Chicago Press.

Marshall, Grant N., Ron D. Hays, Cathy D. Sherbourne, and Kenneth B. Wells. 1993. "The Structure of Patient Satisfaction with Outpatient Medical Care." *Psychological Assessment* 5(4):477–483.

Mass, James W. 1975. "Biogenic Amines and Depression: Biochemical and Pharmacological Separation of Two Types of Depression." *Archives of General Psychiatry* 32:1357–1361.

Massaro, Thomas A., Jiri Nemec, and Ivan Kalman. 1994. "Health System Reform in the Czech Republic: Policy Lessons from the Initial Experience of the General Health Insurance Company." *Journal of the American Medical Association* 271(23):1870–1874.

McClellan, Mark. 1995. "Uncertainty, Health-Care Technologies, and Health Care Choices." *American Economic Review* 85(2):38–44.

McClellan, Mark, Barbara J. McNeil, and Joseph P. Newhouse. 1994. "Does More Intensive Treatment of Acute Myocardial Infarction in the Elderly Reduce Mortality? Analysis Using Instrumental Variables." *Journal of the American Medical Association* 272(11):859–866.

McGuire, Thomas G. 1993. *The Relationship among Coverage, Access to Services, and Health Outcomes: Case Study of Depression.* Paper prepared under contract H3/6690.1 from the Office of Technology Assessment.

McHorney, Colleen, John E. Ware, Jr., J. F. Rachel Lu, and Cathy D. Sherbourne. 1994. "The MOS 36-Item Short-Form Health Survey (SF-36): III. Tests of Data Quality, Scaling Assumptions, and Reliability across Diverse Patient Groups." *Medical Care* 32(1):40–66.

McHorney, Colleen, John E. Ware, Jr., and Anastasia E. Raczek. 1993. "The MOS 36-Item Short-Form Health Survey (SF-36): II. Psychometric and Clinical Tests of Validity in Measuring Physical and Mental Health Constructs." *Medical Care* 31(3):247–263.

McHorney, Colleen A., John E. Ware, Jr., William Rogers, Anastasia E. Raczek, and J. F. Rachel Lu. 1992. "The Validity and Relative Precision of MOS Short- and Long-Form Health Status Scales and Dartmouth COOP Charts: Results from the Medical Outcomes Study." *Medical Care* 30 (5 Suppl):MS253–265.

Mechanic, David, Ronald Angel, and Lorraine Davies. 1991. "Risk and Selection Processes between the General and the Specialty Mental Health Sectors." *Journal of Health and Social Behavior* 32(1):49–64.

Mendelson, Myer. 1992. "Psychodynamics." In Eugene S. Paykel, ed., *Handbook of Affective Disorders.* New York: The Guilford Press, pp. 195–207.

Meredith, Lisa S., Kenneth B. Wells, and Patricia Camp. 1994. "Clinician Specialty and Treatment Style for Depressed Outpatients with and without Medical Comorbidities." *Archives of Family Medicine* 3(12):1065–1072.

Meredith, Lisa S., Kenneth B. Wells, Sherrie H. Kaplan, and Rebecca M. Mazel. 1996. "Counseling Typically Provided for Depression: Role of Clinician Specialty and Payment System." *Archives of General Psychiatry.*

Meyer, Bruce D., 1995. "Natural and Quasi-Experiments in Economics." *Journal of Business and Economic Statistics* 13:151–162.

Mezzich, Juan E., Gerald A. Coffman, and Shelley M. Goodpastor. 1982. "A Format for DSM-III Diagnostic Formulation—Experience with 1,111 Consecutive Patients." *American Journal of Psychiatry* 139(5):591–596.

Mills, James L. 1993. "Data Torturing." *New England Journal of Medicine* 329:1196–1199.

Mintz, Jim, Lois Imber Mintz, Mary Jane Arruda, and Sue Sook Hwang. 1992. "Treatments of Depression and the Functional Capacity to Work." *Archives of General Psychiatry* 49(10):761–768.

Miranda, Jeanne, Ann A. Hohmann, and C. Clifford Attkisson. 1994. "Methodologic Perspective: Getting Answers to the Most Important Questions." In Jeanne Miranda, Ann A. Hohmann, C. Clifford Attkisson, and David B. Larson, eds., *Mental Disorders in Primary Care.* San Francisco, Calif.: Jossey-Bass Publishers, Inc.

Miranda, Jeanne, and Ricardo Muñoz. 1994. "Intervention for Minor Depression in Primary Care Patients." *Psychosomatic Medicine* 56(2):136–141.

Mirowsky, John, and Catherine E. Ross. 1989. "Psychiatric Diagnosis as Reified Measurement." *Journal of Health and Social Behavior* 30(1):11–25.

Mitchell, Jean M., and Kathryn H. Anderson. 1989. "Mental Health and the Labor Force Participation of Older Workers." *Inquiry* 26(2):262–271.

Moos, Rudolf H. 1990. "Depressed Outpatients' Life Contexts, Amount of Treatment, and Treatment Outcome." *Journal of Nervous and Mental Diseases* 178(2):105–112.

Mullahy, John, and Jody L. Sindelar. 1993. "Alcoholism, Work, and Income." *Journal of Labor Economics* 11:494–520.

Mumford, Emily, Herbert J. Schlesinger, Gene V. Glass, Cathleen Patrick, and Timothy Cuerdon. 1984. "A New Look at Evidence about Reduced Cost of Medical Utilization Following Mental Health Treatment." *American Journal of Psychiatry* 141(10):1145–1158.

Muñoz, Richard F., Steven D. Hollon, Ellen McGrath, Lynn P. Rehm, and Gary R. VandenBos. 1994. "On the AHCPR Depression in Primary Care Guidelines: Further Considerations for Practitioners." *American Psychologist* 49(1):42–61.

Murphy, Jane M., Richard R. Monson, Donald C. Olivier, Arthur M. Sobol, and Alexander H. Leighton. 1987. "Affective Disorders and Mortality." *Archives of General Psychiatry* 44(5):473–480.

Myers, Jerome K., Myrna M. Weissman, Gary L. Tischler, Charles E. Holzer III, Philip J. Leaf, Helen Orvaschel, James C. Anthony, Jeffrey H. Boyd, Jock D. Burke, Jr., Morton Kramer, and Roger Stoltzman. 1984. "Six-Month Prevalence of Psychiatric Disorders in Three Communities." *Archives of General Psychiatry* 41(10):959–967.

Narrow, William E., Darrel A. Regier, Donald S. Rae, Ronald W. Manderscheid, and Ben Z. Locke. 1993. "Use of Services by Persons with Mental and Addictive Disorders: Findings from the National Institute of Mental Health Epidemiologic Catchment Area Program." *Archives of General Psychiatry* 50(2):95–107.

Neuhaus, John M. 1992. "Statistical Methods for Longitudinal and Clustered Designs with Binary Responses." *Statistical Methods in Medical Research* 1:249–273.

Newhouse, Joseph P., and the Insurance Experiment Group. 1993. *Free for All? Lessons from the RAND Health Insurance Experiment.* Cambridge, Mass.: Harvard University Press.

Nielsen, Arthur C., and Thomas A. Williams. 1980. "Depression in Ambulatory Medical Patients: Prevalence by Self-Report Questionnaire and Recognition by Nonpsychiatric Physicians." *Archives of General Psychiatry* 37(9):999–1004.

NIH Consensus Development Panel on Depression in Late Life. 1992. "Diagnosis and Treatment of Depression in Late Life." *Journal of the American Medical Association* 268(8):1018–1024.

Norquist, Grayson S., and Kenneth B. Wells. 1991. "How Do HMOs Reduce Outpatient Mental Health Care Costs?" *American Journal of Psychiatry* 148(1):96–101.

Nurnberger, John I., and Elliot S. Gershon. 1992. "Genetics." In Eugene S. Paykel, ed., *Handbook of Affective Disorders.* New York: The Guilford Press, pp. 131–148.

Olfson, Mark, and Gerald L. Klerman. 1992. "The Treatment of Depression: Prescribing Practices of Primary Care Physicians and Psychiatrists." *Journal of Family Practice* 35(6):627–635.

——— 1993. "Trends in the Prescription of Psychotropic Medications: The Role of Physician Specialty." *Medical Care* 31(6):559–564.

Olfson, Mark, and Harold A. Pincus. 1994a. "Outpatient Psychotherapy in the United States. I. Volume, Costs, and User Characteristics." *American Journal of Psychiatry* 151(9):1281–1288.

——— 1994b. "Outpatient Psychotherapy in the United States, II. Patterns of Utilization." *American Journal of Psychiatry* 151(9):1289–1294.

Oren, Dan A., and Norman E. Rosenthal. 1992. "Seasonal Affective Disorders." In Eugene S. Paykel, ed., *Handbook of Affective Disorders.* Second Edition, pp. 551–567.

Orleans, C. Tracy, Linda K. George, Jeffrey L. Houpt, H. Keith H. Brodie. 1985. "How Primary Care Physicians Treat Psychiatric Disorders: A National Survey of Family Practitioners." *American Journal of Psychiatry* 142(1):52–57.

Ormel, Johan, and J. A. Costa e Silva. 1995. "The Impact of Psychopathology on Disability and Health Perceptions." In T. B. Üstün and N. Sartorius, *Mental Illness in General Health Care: An International Study.* New York: John Wiley and Sons, pp. 335–346.

Ormel, Johan, Maarten W. J. Koeter, Wim Van den Brink, and G. Van de Willige. 1991. "Recognition, Management, and Course of Anxiety and

Depression in General Practice." *Archives of General Psychiatry* 48(8):700–706.

Ormel, Johan, Michael Von Korff, Wim Van den Brink, Wayne Katon, Els Brilman, and Tineke Oldehinkel. 1993. "Depression, Anxiety, and Social Disability Show Synchrony of Change in Primary Care Patients: A 3-1/2 Year Longitudinal Study in Primary Care." *American Journal of Public Health* 83(3):385–390.

Paykel, Eugene S., and Zafra Cooper. 1992. "Life Events and Social Stress." In Eugene S. Paykel, ed., *Handbook of Affective Disorders.* New York: The Guilford Press, pp. 149–170.

Petchey, Roland. 1987. "Health Maintenance Organizations: Just What the Doctor Ordered?" *Journal of Social Policy* 16(4):489–507.

Philipp, Michael, Wolfgang Maier, and Cynthia D. Delmo. 1991a. "The Concept of Major Depression. II. Agreement between Six Competing Operational Definitions in Six Hundred Psychiatric Inpatients." *European Archives of Psychiatry and Clinical Neuroscience* 240(4–5):266–271.

——— 1991b. "The Concept of Major Depression. III. Concurrent Validity of Six Competing Operational Definitions for the Clinical ICD-9 Diagnosis." *European Archives of Psychiatry and Clinical Neuroscience* 240(4–5):272–278.

Popkin, Michael K., Allan L. Callies, and Thomas B. MacKenzie. 1985. "The Outcome of Antidepressant Use in the Medically Ill." *Archives of General Psychiatry* 42(12):1160–1163.

Potts, Marilyn K., Marcia Daniels, M. A. Berman, and Kenneth B. Wells. 1990. "A Structured Interview Version of the Hamilton Depression Rating Scale: Evidence of Reliability and Versatility of Administration." *Journal of Psychiatric Research* 24(4):335–350.

Radecki, S. E., and Robert C. Mendenhall. 1986. "Patient Counseling by Primary Care Physicians: Results of a Nationwide Survey." *Patient Education and Counseling* 8(2):165–177.

Rado, S. 1928. "Das Problem der Melancholie." *Int Zeitschr f Psychoanaly* 13. Trans. in *International Journal of Psychoanalysis* 9:420–438.

Regier, Darrel A., Mary E. Farmer, Donald S. Rae, Ben Z. Locke, Samuel J. Keith, Lewis L. Judd, and Frederick K. Goodwin. 1990. "Comorbidity of Mental Disorders with Alcohol and Other Drug Abuse: Results from the Epidemiologic Catchment Area (ECA) Study." *Journal of the American Medical Association* 264(19):2511–2518.

Regier, Darrel A., Irving D. Goldberg, and Carl A. Taube. 1978. "The De Facto U.S. Mental Health Services System." *Archives of General Psychiatry* 35(6):685–693.

Regier, Darrel A., William E. Narrow, Donald S. Rae, Ronald W. Manderscheid, Ben Z. Locke, and Frederick K. Goodwin. 1993. "The De Facto U.S. Mental and Addictive Disorder Service System: Epidemiologic Catchment Area Prospective One-Year Prevalence Rates of Disorders and Services." *Archives of General Psychiatry* 50(2):85–94.

Rice, Dorothy P., Sander Kelman, Leonard S. Miller, and Sarah Dunmeyer. 1990. *The Economic Costs of Alcohol and Drug Abuse and Mental Illness. 1985.* DHHS Publication no. ADM 90–1694. Rockville, Md.: Alcohol, Drug Abuse, and Mental Health Administration.

Rice, Dorothy P., and Leonard D. Miller. 1993. "The Economic Burden of Affective Disorders." *Advances in Health Economics and Health Services Research* 14:37–53. Greenwich, Conn.: JAI Press.

Rice, Thomas, Jon Gabel, Stephen Mick, Clare Lippert, and Colleen Dowd. 1990. "Continuity and Change in Preferred Provider Organizations." *Health Policy* 16:1–18.

Robbins, James M., Laurence J. Kirmayer, Pascal Cathbras, Mark J. Yaffe, Michael Doorkind. 1994. "Physician Characteristics and the Recognition of Depression and Anxiety in Primary Care." *Medical Care* 32:795–812.

Robbins, Trevor W., Eileen M. Joyce, and Barbara J. Sahakian. 1992. "Neuropsychology and Imaging." In Eugene S. Paykel, ed., *Handbook of Affective Disorders.* New York: The Guilford Press, pp. 289–309.

Robins, Lee N., John E. Helzer, Jack Croughan, and Kathryn S. Ratcliff. 1981. "National Institute of Mental Health Diagnostic Interview Schedule: Its History, Characteristics, and Validity." *Archives of General Psychiatry* 38(4):381–389.

Robinson, Leslie A., Jeffrey S. Berman, Robert A. Meimeyer. 1990. "Psychotherapy for the Treatment of Depression: A Comprehensive Review of Controlled Outcome Research." *Psychological Bulletin* 108(1):30–49.

Rodin, Gary, John Craven, and Christine Littlefield. 1991. *Depression in the Medically Ill: An Integrated Approach.* New York: Brunner / Mazel, pp. 7–102.

Rogers, William H., Elizabeth A. McGlynn, Sandra H. Berry, Eugene C. Nelson, Edwin Perrin, Michael Zubkoff, Sheldon Greenfield, Kenneth B. Wells, Anita L. Stewart, Sharon B. Arnold, and John E. Ware, Jr. 1992. "Methods of Sampling." In Anita L. Stewart and John E. Ware, Jr., eds., *Measuring Functioning and Well-Being: The Medical Outcomes Study Approach.* Durham, N.C.: Duke University Press, pp. 27–47.

Rogers, William H., Kenneth B. Wells, Lisa S. Meredith, Roland Sturm, and Audrey Burnam. 1993. "Outcomes for Adult Outpatients with Depression under Prepaid or Fee-for-Service Financing." *Archives of General Psychiatry* 50(7):517–525.

Rosenblatt, Roger A., Daniel C. Cherkin, Ronald Schneeweiss, and L. Gary

Hart. 1983. "The Content of Ambulatory Medical Care in the United States: An Interspecialty Comparison." *New England Journal of Medicine* 309(15):892–897.

Rosenstock, Irwin M. 1974. "Historical Origins of the Health Belief Model." *Health Education Monographs* 2:1–328.

Rost, K., G. R. Smith, B. Guise, and D. Matthews. 1994. "The Deliberate Misdiagnosis of Major Depression in Primary Care." *Archives of Family Medicine* 3:333–337.

Ruhm, Christopher J. 1992. "The Effects of Physical and Mental Health on Female Labor Supply." In Richard G. Frank and Willard G. Manning, Jr., eds., *Economics and Mental Health.* Baltimore, Md.: Johns Hopkins University Press, pp. 152–181.

Sargeant, J. Kent, Martha L. Bruce, Louis P. Florio, and Myrna M. Weissman. 1990. "Factors Associated with One-Year Outcome of Major Depression in the Community." *Archives of General Psychiatry* 47(6):519–526.

Schuckit, Marc A. 1986. "Genetic and Clinical Implications of Alcoholism and Affective Disorder." *American Journal of Psychiatry* 143(2):140–147.

Schulberg, Herbert C., Maureen McClelland, and Barbara J. Burns. 1987. "Depression and Physical Illness: The Prevalence, Causation, and Diagnosis of Comorbidity." *Clinical Psychology Review* 7(2):145–167.

Schulberg, Herbert C., Marjorie Saul, Maureen McClelland, Mary Ganguli, Wallace Christy, and Richard Frank. 1985. "Assessing Depression in Primary Medical and Psychiatric Practices." *Archives of General Psychiatry* 42(12):1164–1170.

Schurman, Rachel A., Janet B. Mitchell, and Peter D. Kramer. 1985. "When Doctors Listen: Counseling Patterns of Nonpsychiatrist Physicians." *American Journal of Psychiatry* 142(8):934–938.

Scott, A. I., and C. P. Freeman. 1992. "Edinburgh Primary Care Depression Study: Treatment Outcome, Patient Satisfaction, and Cost after Sixteen Weeks" [see comments]. *British Medical Journal* 304(6831):833–837.

Seligman, Martin E. P. 1975. *Helplessness: On Depression, Development, and Death.* San Francisco, Calif.: W. H. Freeman.

Shapiro, Sam, Pearl S. German, Elizabeth A. Skinner, Michael Von Korff, Raymond Turner, Lawrence E. Klein, Mark Teitelbaum, Morton Kramer, Jack D. Burke, Jr., and Barbara J. Burns. 1987. "An Experiment to Change Detection and Management of Mental Morbidity in Primary Care." *Medical Care* 25(4):327–339.

Sherbourne, Cathy D. 1992a. "Pain Measures." In Anita L. Stewart and John E. Ware, Jr., eds., *Measuring Functioning and Well-Being: The Medical Outcomes Study Approach.* Durham, N.C.: Duke University Press, pp. 220–234.

—— 1992b. "Social Functioning: Sexual Problems Measures." In Anita L. Stewart and John E. Ware, Jr., eds., *Measuring Functioning and Well-Being: The Medical Outcomes Study Approach.* Durham, N.C.: Duke University Press, pp. 194–204.

—— 1992c. "Social Functioning: Social Activity Limitations Measure." In Anita L. Stewart and John E. Ware, Jr., eds., *Measuring Functioning and Well-Being: The Medical Outcomes Study Approach.* Durham, N.C.: Duke University Press, pp. 173–181.

Sherbourne, Cathy D., Harris M. Allen, Caren J. Kamberg, and Kenneth B. Wells. 1992. "Physical / Psychophysiologic Symptoms Measure." In Anita L. Stewart and John E. Ware, Jr., eds., *Measuring Functioning and Well-Being: The Medical Outcomes Study Approach.* Durham, N.C.: Duke University Press, pp. 260–277.

Sherbourne, Cathy D., and Ronald D. Hays. 1990. "Marital Status, Social Support, and Health Transitions in Chronic Disease Patients." *Journal of Health and Social Behavior* 31(4):328–343.

Sherbourne, Cathy D., Ronald D. Hays, and Kenneth B. Wells. 1995. "Risk Factors for Physical and Mental Health Outcomes and Course of Depression among Depressed Outpatients." *Journal of Clinical and Consulting Psychology* 63(6):345–355.

Sherbourne, Cathy D., Ronald D. Hays, Kenneth B. Wells, William H. Rogers, and M. Audrey Burnam. 1993. "Prevalence of Comorbid Alcohol Disorder and Consumption in Medically Ill and Depressed Patients." *Archives of Family Medicine* 2(11):1142–1150.

Sherbourne, Cathy D., and Caren J. Kamberg. 1992. "Social Functioning: Family and Marital Functioning Measures." In Anita L. Stewart and John E. Ware, Jr., eds., *Measuring Functioning and Well-Being: The Medical Outcomes Study Approach.* Durham, N.C.: Duke University Press, pp. 182–193.

Sherbourne, Cathy D., Anita L. Stewart, and Kenneth B. Wells. 1992. "Role Functioning Measures." In Anita L. Stewart and John E. Ware, Jr., eds., *Measuring Functioning and Well-Being: The Medical Outcomes Study Approach.* Durham, N.C.: Duke University Press, pp. 205–219.

Sherbourne, Cathy D., Kenneth B. Wells, Ronald D. Hays, William H. Rogers, Audrey Burnam, and Lewis L. Judd. 1994. "Subthreshold Depression and Depressive Disorder." *American Journal of Psychiatry* 151(12):1777–1784.

Simon, Gregory E., and Michael Von Korff. 1992. "Reevaluation of Secular Trends in Depression Rates." *American Journal of Epidemiology* 135(12):1411–1422.

Simon, Gregory E., Michael Von Korff, Edward H. Wagner, and William

Barlow. 1993. "Patterns of Antidepressant Use in Community Practice." *General Hospital Psychiatry* 15:399–408.

Simon, Gregory E., Edward Wagner, and Michael Von Korff. 1995. "Cost-Effectiveness Comparisons Using Real World Randomized Trials: The Case of New Antidepressant Drugs." *Journal of Clinical Epidemiology* 48(3):363–373.

Simons, Anne, Judith S. Gordon, Scott M. Monroe, and Michael E. Thase. 1995. "Toward an Integration of Psychologic, Social, and Biologic Factors in Depression: Effects on Outcome and Course of Cognitive Therapy." *Journal of Consulting and Clinical Psychology* 63(3):369–377.

Sireling, Lester I., P. Freeling, Eugene S. Paykel, and B. M. Rao. 1985. "Depression in General Practice: Clinical Features and Comparison with Out-Patients." *British Journal of Psychiatry* 147:119–126.

Smith, Angela L., and Myrna M. Weissman. 1992. "Epidemiology." In Eugene S. Paykel, ed., *Handbook of Affective Disorders*. New York: The Guilford Press, pp. 111–129.

Spaner, D., R. C. Bland, and S. C. Newman. 1994. "Major Depressive Disorder." *Acta Psychiatrica Scandinavia.* Suppl 376:7–15.

Stewart, Anita L. 1990. "Psychometric Considerations in Functional Status Instruments." In Michael Lipkin, ed., *Functional Status Measurement in Primary Care*. New York: Springer-Verlag.

Stewart, Anita L., Ronald D. Hays, and John E. Ware, Jr. 1988. "The MOS Short-Form General Health Survey: Reliability and Validity in a Patient Population." *Medical Care* 26(7):724–735.

———— 1992. "Health Perceptions, Energy / Fatigue, and Health Distress Measures." In Anita L. Stewart and John E. Ware, Jr., eds., *Measuring Functioning and Well-Being: The Medical Outcomes Study Approach.* Durham, N.C.: Duke University Press, pp. 143–172.

Stewart, Anita L., and Caren J. Kamberg. 1992. "Physical Functioning Measures." In Anita L. Stewart and John E. Ware, Jr., eds., *Measuring Functioning and Well-Being: The Medical Outcomes Study Approach.* Durham, N.C.: Duke University Press, pp. 86–101.

Stewart, Anita L., Cathy D. Sherbourne, Kenneth B. Wells, M. Audrey Burnam, William H. Rogers, Ronald D. Hays, and John E. Ware, Jr. 1993. "Do Depressed Patients in Different Treatment Settings Have Different Levels of Well-Being and Functioning?" *Journal of Consulting and Clinical Psychology* 61(5):849–857.

Stewart, Anita L., and John E. Ware, Jr., eds. 1992. *Measuring Functioning and Well-Being: The Medical Outcomes Study Approach.* Durham, N.C.: Duke University Press.

Stewart, Anita L., John E. Ware, Jr., Cathy D. Sherbourne, and Kenneth B. Wells. 1992. "Psychological Distress / Well-Being and Cognitive Functioning Measures." In Anita L. Stewart and John E. Ware, Jr., eds., *Measuring Functioning and Well-Being: The Medical Outcomes Study Approach.* Durham, N.C.: Duke University Press, pp. 102–142.

Stoudemire, Alan, Richard Frank, Nancy Hedemark, Mark Kamlet, and Dan Blazer. 1986. "The Economic Burden of Depression." *General Hospital Psychiatry* 8(6):387–394.

Sturm, Roland, Catherine Jackson, Lisa S. Meredith, Winnie Yip, Willard G. Manning, William H. Rogers, and Kenneth B. Wells. 1995. "Mental Health Care Utilization in Prepaid and Fee-for-Service Plans among Depressed Patients in the Medical Outcomes Study." *Health Services Research* 30:319–340.

Sturm, Roland, Elizabeth McGlynn, Lisa S. Meredith, Kenneth B. Wells, Willard G. Manning, and William H. Rogers. 1994. "Switches between Prepaid and Fee-for-Service Health Systems among Depressed Outpatients: Results from the Medical Outcomes Study." *Medical Care* 32:917–929.

Sturm, Roland, Lisa S. Meredith, and Kenneth B. Wells. Forthcoming. "Provider Choice and Continuity for the Treatment of Depression." *Medical Care.*

Sturm, Roland, and Kenneth B. Wells. 1995. "How Can Care for Depression Become More Cost-Effective?" *Journal of the American Medical Association* 273(1):51–58.

Styron, William. 1992. *Darkness Visible: A Memoir of Madness.* New York: First Vintage Books, p. 84.

Swarz, Marvin, Bernard Carroll, and Dan G. Blazer. 1989. "In Response to Psychiatric Diagnosis as Reified Measurement: An Invited Comment on Mirowsky and Ross." *Journal of Health and Social Behavior* 30(1):33–34.

Swindle, Ralph W., Ruth C. Cronkite, and Rudolf H. Moos. 1989. "Life Stressors, Social Resources, Coping, and the Four-Year Course of Unipolar Depression." *Journal of Abnormal Psychology* 98(4):468–477.

Tarlov, Alvin R., John E. Ware, Jr., Sheldon Greenfield, Eugene C. Nelson, Edwin Perrin, and Michael Zubkoff. 1989. "Medical Outcomes Study: An Application of Methods for Monitoring the Results of Medical Care." *Journal of the American Medical Association* 262(7):925–930.

Task Force on DSM-IV. 1994. *Diagnostic and Statistical Manual of Mental Disorders. Fourth Edition (DSM-IV).* Washington, D.C.: American Psychiatric Association.

Torrance, George. 1986. "Measurement of Health State Utilities for Economic Appraisal." *Journal of Health Economics* 5:1–30.

Tweed, Daniel L., and Linda K. George. 1989. "A More Balanced Perspective on Psychiatric Diagnosis as Reified Measurement: An Invited Comment on Mirowsky and Ross." *Journal of Health and Social Behavior* 30(1):35–37.

U.S. Bureau of the Census. 1994. *Statistical Abstract of the United States: 1994.* 114th ed. Washington, D.C., pp. 92–101.

Üstün, T. B., and N. Norman, eds. 1995. Mental Illness in General Health Care: An International Study. New York: John Wiley and Sons.

Üstün, T. B., N. Sartorius, J. A. Costa e Silva, David Goldberg, Y. Lecrubier, Johan Ormel, Michael Von Korgg, and Hans-Ulrich Wittchen. 1995. "Conclusions." In *Mental Illness in General Health Care: An International Study.* New York: John Wiley and Sons, pp. 371–376.

Üstün, T. B., and M. Von Korff. 1995. "Primary Mental Health Services: Access and Provision of Care." In *Mental Illness in General Health Care: An International Study.* New York: John Wiley and Sons.

Van den Brink, Wim, Anne Leenstra, Johan Ormel, and Gerard van de Willige. 1991. "Mental Health Intervention Programs in Primary Care: Their Scientific Basis." *Journal of Affective Disorders.* 21(4):273–284.

Von Korff, Michael, Johan Ormel, Wayne Katon, and Elizabeth H. B. Lin. 1992. "Disability and Depression among High Utilizers of Health Care: A Longitudinal Analysis." *Archives of General Psychiatry* 49(2):91–100.

Von Korff, Michael, Sam Shapiro, Jack D. Burke, Mark Teitlebaum, Elizabeth A. Skinner, Pearl German, Raymond W. Turner, Lawrence Klein, and Barbara Burns. 1987. "Anxiety and Depression in a Primary Care Clinic." *Archives of General Psychiatry* 44(2):152–156.

Von Korff, Michael, and Gregory E. Simon. 1994. "Methodologic Perspective: Getting Answers to the Most Important Questions." In Jeanne Miranda, Ann A. Hohmann, C. Clifford Attkisson, and David B. Larson, eds., *Mental Disorders in Primary Care.* San Francisco, Calif.: Jossey-Bass Publishers, Inc.

Ware, John E., Jr. 1984. "Methodological Considerations in the Selection of Health Status Assessment Procedures." In Nanette K. Wenger, Margaret E. Mattson, Curt D. Furberg, and Jack Elinson, eds., *Assessment of Quality of Life in Clinical Trials of Cardiovascular Therapies.* New York: Le Jacq Publishing, Inc., pp. 87–111.

—— 1986. "The Assessment of Health Status." In Linda H. Aiken and David Mechanic, eds., *Applications of Social Sciences to Clinical Medicine and Health Policy.* New Brunswick, N.J.: Rutgers University Press, pp. 204–228.

—— 1992. "Measures for a New Era of Health Assessment." In Anita L. Stewart and John E. Ware, Jr., eds., *Measuring Functioning and Well-Being: The Medical Outcomes Study Approach.* Durham, N.C.: Duke University Press, pp. 1–11.

———— 1993a. "Measuring Patients' Views: The Optimum Outcome Measure." *British Medical Journal* 306(6890):1429–1430.

———— 1993b. *SF-36 Health Survey: Manual and Interpretation Guide.* Boston, Mass.: The Health Institute, New England Medical Center.

Ware, John E., Jr., and Cathy D. Sherbourne. 1992. "The MOS 36-Item Short-Form Health Survey (SF-36): I. Conceptual Framework and Item Selection." *Medical Care* 30(6):473–483.

Ware, John E., Jr., Cathy D. Sherbourne, and Allyson R. Davies. 1992. "Developing and Testing the MOS 20-Item Short-Form Health Survey: A General Population Application." In Anita L. Stewart and John E. Ware, Jr., eds., *Measuring Functioning and Well-Being: The Medical Outcomes Study Approach.* Durham, N.C.: Duke University Press, pp. 277–290.

Ware, John E., Jr., Mark Kosinski, and Susan D. Keller. 1994. *SF-36 Physical and Mental Health Summary Scales: A User's Manual.* Boston, Mass.: The Health Institute.

Weissman, Myrna M., and Gerald L. Klerman. 1992. "Depression: Current Understanding and Changing Trends." *Annual Review of Public Health* 13:319–339.

Weissman, Myrna M., Philip J. Leaf, Gary L. Tischler, Dan G. Blazer, Marvin Karno, Martha Livingston Bruce, and Louis P. Florio. 1988. "Affective Disorders in Five United States Communities." *Psychological Medicine* 18(1):141–153.

Weissman, Myrna M., Jerome K. Myers, and W. Douglas Thompson. 1981. "Depression and Its Treatment in a U.S. Urban Community: 1975–1976." *Archives of General Psychiatry* 38(4):417–421.

Wells, Kenneth B. 1985. *Depression as a Tracer Condition for the National Study of Medical Care Outcomes.* Publication no. R-3293-RWJ / HJK. Santa Monica, Calif.: RAND.

Wells, Kenneth B., Boris M. Astrachan, Gary L. Tischler, and Jürgen Ünützer. 1995. "Issues and Approaches in Evaluating Managed Mental Health Care." *The Milbank Quarterly* 73(1):57–75.

Wells, Kenneth B., M. Audrey Burnam, William Rogers, and Patti Camp. 1995. "Severity of Depression in Prepaid and Fee-for-Service General Medical and Mental Health Specialty Practices." *Medical Care* 33(4):350–364.

Wells, Kenneth B., M. Audrey Burnam, William Rogers, Ron Hays, and Patti Camp. 1992. "The Course of Depression in Adult Outpatients: Results from the Medical Outcomes Study." *Archives of General Psychiatry* 49(10):788–794.

Wells, Kenneth B., Jacqueline Golding, and M. Audrey Burnam. 1988. "Psychiatric Disorder and Limitations in Physical Functioning in a

Sample of the Los Angeles General Population." *American Journal of Psychiatry* 145(6):712–717.

Wells, Kenneth B., Ronald D. Hays, M. Audrey Burnam, William Rogers, Sheldon Greenfield, and John E. Ware, Jr. 1989. "Detection of Depressive Disorder for Patients Receiving Prepaid or Fee-for-Service Care: Results from the Medical Outcomes Study." *Journal of the American Medical Association* 262(23):3298–3302.

Wells, Kenneth B., Wayne Katon, Bill Rogers, and Patti Camp. 1994. "Use of Minor Tranquilizers and Antidepressant Medications by Depressed Outpatients: Results from the Medical Outcomes Study." *American Journal of Psychiatry* 151(5):694–700.

Wells, Kenneth B., Charles E. Lewis, Barbara Leake, Mary Kay Schleiter, and Robert H. Brook. 1986. "The Practices of General and Subspecialty Internists in Counseling about Smoking and Exercise." *American Journal of Public Health* 76(8):1009–1013.

Wells, Kenneth B., Willard G. Manning, Jr., and Bernadette Benjamin. 1986. "Use of Outpatient Mental Health Services in HMO and Fee-for-Service Plans: Results from a Randomized Controlled Trial." *Health Services Research* 21:453–474.

Wells, Kenneth B., Willard G. Manning, Jr., M. Audrey Burnam, Sheldon Greenfield, and John E. Ware, Jr. 1991. "How the Medical Comorbidity of Depressed Patients Differs across Health Care Settings: Results from the Medical Outcomes Study." *American Journal of Psychiatry* 148(12):1688–1696.

Wells, Kenneth B., Willard G. Manning, Jr., Naihua Duan, Joseph P. Newhouse, and John E. Ware, Jr. 1987. "Cost-Sharing and the Use of General Medical Physicians for Outpatient Mental Health Care." *Health Services Research* 22(1):1–18.

Wells, Kenneth B., Willard G. Manning, Jr., and R. Burciaga Valdez. 1989. "The Effects of Insurance Generosity on the Psychological Distress and Psychological Well-Being of a General Population." *Archives of General Psychiatry* 46:315–321.

——— 1990. "The Effects of a Prepaid Group Practice on Mental Health Outcomes." *Health Services Research* 25(4):615–624.

Wells, Kenneth B., Anita L. Stewart, Ronald D. Hays, M. Audrey Burnam, William Rogers, Marcia Daniels, Sandra Berry, Sheldon Greenfield, and John E. Ware, Jr. 1989. "The Functioning and Well-Being of Depressed Patients: Results from the Medical Outcomes Study." *Journal of the American Medical Association* 262(7):914–949.

Wells, Kenneth B., John E. Ware, Jr., and Charles E. Lewis. 1984a. "Physicians' Practices in Counseling Patients about Health Habits." *Medical Care* 22(3):240–246.

——— 1984b. "Physicians' Attitudes in Counseling Patients about Smoking." *Medical Care* 22(4):240–246.

Wender, Paul H., Seymour S. Kety, David Rosenthal, Fini Schulsinger, Jorgen Ortmann, and Inge Lunde. 1986. "Psychiatric Disorders in the Biological and Adoptive Families of Adopted Individuals with Affective Disorders." *Archives of General Psychiatry* 43(10):923–929.

White, Halbert J. 1982. "Instrumental Variables Regression with Independent Observations." *Econometrica* 50:483–499.

WHO Mental Health Collaborating Centres. 1989. "Pharmacotherapy of Depressive Disorders: A Consensus Statement." *Journal of Affective Disorders* 17(2):197–198.

Wickramaratne, Priya J., Myrna M. Weissman, Philip J. Leaf, and Theodore R. Holford. 1989. "Age, Period, and Cohort Effects on the Risk of Major Depression: Results from Five United States Communities." *Journal of Clinical Epidemiology* 42(4):333–343.

Wilhelm, Kay, and Gordon Parker. 1994. "Sex Differences in Lifetime Depression Rates: Fact or Artifact?" *Psychological Medicine* 24(1):97–111.

Willner, Paul. 1995. "Dopaminergic Mechanisms in Depression and Mania." In Floyd Bloom and David Kupfer, eds., *Psychopharmacology: The Fourth Generation of Progress*. New York: Raven Press, pp. 921–932.

Winokur, George, William Coryell, Martin Keller, Jean Endicott, and Andrew Leon. 1995. "A Family Study of Manic-Depressive (Bipolar I) Disease: Is It a Distinct Illness Separable from Primary Unipolar Depression?" *Archives of General Psychiatry* 52(5):367–373.

World Bank. 1987. *Financing Health Care in Developing Countries*. Washington, D.C.: World Bank Policy Study.

——— 1993. *Investing in Health*. New York: Oxford University Press.

World Health Organization. 1948. "World Health Organization Constitution." In *Basic Documents*. Geneva: World Health Organization.

——— 1990. *Mental and Behavioral Disorders*. Geneva: World Health Organization.

——— 1991. Tenth Revision of the International Classification of Diseases, Chapter V: Mental and Behavioral Disorders (including disorders of psychological development). Geneva: World Health Organization, Division of Mental Health.

Wright, Alastair F. 1994. "Should General Practitioners Be Testing for Depression?" *British Journal of General Practice* 44(380):132–135.

Zung, William W. K., W. Eugene Broadhead, and Mary E. Roth. 1993. "Prevalence of Depressive Symptoms in Primary Care." *Journal of Family Practice* 37(4):337–344.

Index